House Officer Guide to ICU Care

Fundamentals of Management of the Heart and Lungs

Second Edition

House Officer Guide to ICU Care

Fundamentals of Management of the Heart and Lungs

Second Edition

John A. Elefteriades, M.D.
Professor of Surgery
Director of Adult Cardiac Procedures
Yale University School of Medicine
New Haven, Connecticut

Alexander S. Geha, M.D.
Professor of Surgery
Chief, Division of Cardiothoracic Surgery
Case Western Reserve School of Medicine
Cleveland, Ohio

Lawrence S. Cohen, M.D.
The Ebenezer K. Hunt Professor of Medicine
Deputy Dean
Yale University School of Medicine
New Haven, Connecticut

Foreword by Burton E. Sobel, M.D.

RAVEN PRESS ❧ **NEW YORK**

Raven Press, Ltd., 1185 Avenue of the Americas, New York, New York 10036

Made in the United States of America

Library of Congress Cataloging-in-Publication Data

Elefteriades, John A.
    House officer guide to ICU care : fundamentals of management of the heart and lungs / John A. Elefteriades, Alexander S. Geha, Lawrence S. Cohen ; foreword by Burton E. Sobel.—2nd ed.
        p.   cm.
    Includes bibliographical references and index.
    ISBN 0-7817-0198-8
    1. Cardiac intensive care.   2. Respiratory intensive care.   3. Surgical intensive care.   I. Geha, Alexander S. (Alexander Salim), 1936–   .   II. Cohen, Lawrence S.   III. Title.   IV. Title: House officer guide to intensive care unit care.
    [DNLM: 1. Thoracic Surgery.   2. Heart Surgery.   3. Intensive Care Units.   4. Postoperative Care.   WF 980 E38h 1994]
    RC684.C36E44   1994
    616.1'2028—dc20
    DNLM/DLC
    for Library of Congress   94-6124

9 8 7 6 5 4 3 2 1

To our families
for their continued understanding

Contents

Acknowledgments

The authors would like to express appreciation to the following individuals for their work on the First Edition: Mary Samokar for expert secretarial and administrative work, Marjorie Nelson of University Park Press for originating the project, Michael Treadway of University Park Press for organizing, editing, and clarifying the text, Drs. Lawrence S. Cohen, Paul G. Barash, and James Biondi of Yale University School of Medicine for reviewing and criticizing the manuscript, and Dwight C. McGoon for his thoughtful Foreword.

Important additional acknowledgments for the Second Edition are as follows: Sincere appreciation is expressed to Gail Thomas for her expertise in bringing academic projects to fruition and for her dedication to Yale University; John F. Setaro, Assistant Professor of Medicine (Cardiology), for his excellent chapter on management of acute valvular heart disease; Kevin Johnson of Diagnostic Imaging for providing the illustrative examples of the various modalities of acute cardiac imaging; and Lawrence Solomon and George Cole for their valuable suggestions from the student's perspective. Special appreciation is expressed to Lisa Berger of Raven Press for her invaluable guidance.

Foreword to the
First Edition

It is said that the human brain, given free access to the world's libraries and now also to computer networks, has at its dendritic "fingertips" a capacity for retrieval of some 100,000 trillion bits (binary digits) of information. Surely at least this much information has been processed across the cerebral cortex of most survivors of a medical education, if one takes into account all of their premedical acculturation and intensive postdoctoral training. Such a vast educational investment is not just pedantic overkill, for only through an understanding of the historical and theoretical bases of our knowledge of the complexities of health and disease can the most effective strategies for treatment and prevention, and especially their most effective advancement, become available.

Yet even when steeped in all this academic indoctrination, or perhaps because of it, when the neophyte first (and at long last) assumes some responsibility for a critically sick patient in an intensive care unit, he or she typically experiences a surge of insecurity and self-doubt. All of that massive background of theoretical knowledge, gleaned from texts, articles, lectures, and bits of prior exposure to patient care, suddenly becomes inadequate to deal with the often relatively simple but quintessentially critical moment-to-moment decisions that are unavoidable in the intensive care setting: whether to extubate or not, reoperate for bleeding or not, administer countershock or not, transfuse or not, call in the family or not, etc., etc. There is simply no possibility of moving back to a given branch on the decision tree to test the other choices.

As with any other demanding activity, experience and practice bestow efficiency, accuracy, and self-confidence. Until that welcome milestone is reached, however, the novice to the stressful demands of decision-making in the intensive care setting longs for a plain-talk, bare-bones listing of the variables comprising the algorithms whereby these decisions are reached.

This book succeeds to a surprising degree in achieving such a mission. It provides a condensation of these essential materials that is incapable of further reduction. Its facts and statements are (unlike the preceding comments) presented snappily and crisply in a down-to-business manner.

The challenging dilemma of any teaching program is the safe and efficient transition of the gulf between factual knowledge and its practical application. Acquisition of knowledge at the traditional, expensive school of trial-and-error must be minimized if the "error" component of that curriculum, with its legacy of tragedy and suffering, is to be avoided. A book such as this one would become a travesty if in any way it were used as a procedural manual intended to allow a technician without medical training to manage patients in intensive care. However, as a handbook for the student or house officer who already has a broad knowledge of the basic tenets and theory of medicine, it is surely a most valuable resource.

Dwight C. McGoon, M.D.
Mayo Medical School
Rochester, Minnesota

Foreword

Although "doctor" is derived from the Latin, *docere*, to teach, few doctors of medicine are also gifted teachers. Fortunately, the three authors of this book are teachers in the finest tradition. For students, house officers, generalists, and specialists, all of whom are inundated with an exponentially increasing amount of information, this guide will be invaluable. Intensivists must make decisions expeditiously and implement therapy judiciously for fragile and severely compromised patients. With wisdom predicated on extensive personal experience, the authors of the *House Officer Guide to ICU Care* succeed admirably in identifying the core aspects of problems encountered and provide practical guidelines for optimal diagnosis and treatment.

Archibald MacLeish believed that much antisocial behavior was attributable to an ever-widening gulf between individual members of society and the technologies on which they depend. This book will help to overcome analogous technological alienation of house officers who care for patients with extraordinarily difficult problems requiring sophisticated and complex interventions.

The word "care" in the title is pivotal. The guide is oriented toward the well-being of patients rather than technology for its own sake. Horrific circumstances, witnessed all too often, exemplified by a group of house officers gazing at machines displaying wave forms rather than at a patient who may be apneic, can be best avoided by lessons learned from the guide.

The term "guide" in the title reflects the authors' sensitivity to the importance of medical judgment. It avoids the pitfalls of "algorithmic medicine." The authors empower the reader to chart a course consistent with physiologic principles, astute observation, and practical therapeutics.

This edition follows the first after a nine-year interval. Advances in pathophysiology, diagnosis relying on biochemical markers, and elegant imaging by transesophageal echocardiography and MRI, circulatory-assist devices, "smart" pacemakers and implantable defibrillators, ablation and surgery for the treatment of arrhythmia, and pharmacology with novel anti-arrhythmic, anti-injury, anti-ischemic, vasodilator, and cardiostimulatory agents have been incorporated in a thoroughly rewritten work. Despite its breadth, the information is assimilated readily. The authors' approach of first delineating underlying physiologic principles, then principles underlying therapy, (including pharmacodynamics and operational aspects of devices), and only then describing how the agent or device is used (with specific dose regimens and guidelines for use of equipment) is indeed empowering. The diagrams of wave forms and operational features of complex equipment along with outlines for selection of appropriate therapeutic interventions are particularly helpful.

The book is eminently practical. For example, the authors discuss not only the use of ventilators and novel modes of ventilatory support but also practical aspects of weaning. They consider not only the impact of mechanical ventilation on hemodynamic recordings but also the consequent artifacts that may cloud interpretation. They consider not only electrophysiologic principles underlying arrhythmia but also often-overlooked phenomena, such as inducibility by Swan-Ganz catheters and other devices with a potential for serious mischief.

This guide's thorough reference lists facilitate delving into selected phenomena in depth. Even mundane topics, such as management of chest tube drainage systems and their visual monitoring to detect the physiologic hallmark of serious bleeding, are treated in a thoroughly scholarly fashion.

Perhaps of most importance, the *House Officer Guide to ICU Care* is cohesive. Because the book is written by three knowledgeable clinicians steeped in clinical science and involved daily in the care of patients, it boasts remarkable clarity. The authors support their recommendations rigorously with references to the literature, but it is their collective wisdom that is particularly telling. These three teacher/physicians have made a monumental contribution to the improvement of patient care in an area in which the intelligent use of modern technology increasingly requires sophisticated judgment and expertise predicated on a broad base of knowledge of pathophysiology and therapeutics.

Burton E. Sobel, M.D.
The University of Vermont
College of Medicine
Burlington, Vermont

Preface to the First Edition

This guide is designed to fill the need for a practical manual for the care of critically ill patients. The emphasis is on the postoperative cardiothoracic surgical patient, but nearly all of the information covered is relevant to medical and general surgical patients in intensive care as well.

The various chapters have grown out of lectures given to students and residents rotating through the Cardiothoracic Surgery Service at Yale University School of Medicine. Students and junior house officers have repeatedly emphasized their difficulty in finding written sources for the "hands-on" information contained in this manual. Included are sections that describe the practical use of mechanical intensive care equipment such as face masks, ventilators, pacemakers, the defibrillator, transducers, monitors, the Swan-Ganz catheter, the intra-aortic balloon pump, and chest tubes and drainage systems. Also included are practically oriented chapters on patient management. Treatment of arrhythmias, hemodynamic management, use of inotropes and afterload-reducing agents, management of postoperative bleeding, management of cardiac arrest and near arrest, and treatment of chest trauma are covered. Specific chapters provide a general approach and orientation to problems following noncardiac thoracic surgery, to acute aortic dissection, and to prosthetic heart valves and anticoagulation. Breadth of coverage is restricted largely to the cardiorespiratory systems.

The emphasis throughout this guide is to provide basic knowledge and to outline fundamentals in order to enable the physician starting out in caring for ICU patients to make reasonable management decisions—and to make them independently. At most medical centers, the ICUs are left in the care of junior physicians for significant periods of time when senior personnel are occupied in the operating room or elsewhere. Adherence to the principles outlined in this guide should prevent major errors from being made while junior staff exclusively are at the scene. It is hoped to convey, with this guide, most of what our junior house officers say is the considerable maturity in patient care they acquire while rotating through our Cardiothoracic Surgical Service.

Only our own proven methods of patient care are covered. Patient care patterns do vary from center to center. This guide is meant to provide the house officer with one sound method of handling each major ICU problem that may arise. This one view-point may be expanded or modified as the individual reader gains experience at his particular medical center.

While references to some experimental studies are included, no attempt is made to cover fully the primary experimental evidence behind all management fundamentals presented. At the end of each chapter, following the specific references, a list of selected reading with annotations is appended to guide the interested reader to further, more detailed information.

There exist already numerous comprehensive volumes for the intensive care specialist. The goal of the present guide is to provide an introductory manual that may be mastered in days or weeks in preparation for a particular ICU rotation.

It is hoped that the guide may be of use especially to medical students and junior house officers embarking on ICU responsibilities. The material covered is fundamental enough to be of value as well to intensive care nurses and nurses in training. Physicians' assistants and respiratory therapists, as well, may find the guide useful.

Throughout the text, key concepts are emphasized in bold print to allow easy identification and efficient review. Figures and diagrams are used liberally to amplify the text.

Preface

The changes in the Second Edition fall into two general categories. The first is a thorough updating to reflect changes and advances in ICU care in the nine years since the original publication. The second is an expansion in scope beyond the specific care of the postoperative patient to that of the general care of the heart and lungs in medical as well as surgical patients.

Many new topics have been added to the text to reflect advances in care since the original publication. Arrhythmia surgery has emerged as a major field of endeavor, and a new chapter has been devoted to aspects of care after such operations. A new chapter covers cardiac assist devices that have become additional tools in the armamentarium for management of life-threatening pump failure. Material has been added to existing chapters to cover pressure support ventilation, the use of adenosine for supraventricular arrhythmias, the temporary external DDD pacemaker, changes in recommendations for conduct of cardiopulmonary resuscitation, use of noninvasive oxygen saturation monitors, synergistic use of amrinone and β-agonist inotropic medications, temporary pacing via the Swan-Ganz catheter, new intravenous and oral β-blocking and calcium channel blocking medications, aprotinin, heparin-induced thrombosis and thrombocytopenia, and the importance of the magnesium ion.

We discovered through direct feedback from house officers throughout the country that this text was being used not only by surgical housestaff but also by medical housestaff, including medical interns and residents and cardiology fellows, as well as by specialists in other fields who at times are called upon to care for ICU patients. It is this feedback that inspired the expansion of the scope of the text. Care of the postoperative cardiothoracic patient, the original focus, is still covered thoroughly. In addition, care of the the medical ICU patient is emphasized as well. Much of the original material, such as the ventilator management and the care of arrhythmias, applies equally well to the medical patient. Additional chapters added specifically to expand the scope of the text include those on cardiac imaging in the acutely ill patient (including transthoracic echocardiography, transesophageal echocardiography, nuclear scanning, CAT scanning, and MRI imaging), management of acute coronary ischemia, acute management of valvular heart disease, and management of acute pulmonary disease.

The broadening of scope to include the medical ICU patient is reflected in the invaluable addition of Lawrence S. Cohen as an author of the book.

As in the First Edition, this is an introductory text covering what the house officer absolutely, positively needs to know to feel comfortable and to deliver safe, front-line care—especially during those many times when experienced leadership is not immediately on site.

1 Respirators and Respiratory Management

The management of patients on respirators is a topic that junior house staff often find confusing. Management decisions are quite simple if a few basic principles are clarified and categories of dysfunction are recognized.

The purpose of this chapter is to enable the house officer to manage any respirator problem on any patient. Initial consideration is given to basic physiologic principles regarding oxygenation and ventilation and the assessment of the adequacy and efficiency of these processes. Next, we discuss the practical respiratory parameters that must be set when a patient is first placed on a ventilator. Selection of the initial settings is clarified. Then the categories of dysfunction that may require changes in the initial settings are described, as is the method of changing the initial respirator settings to correct these abnormalities. Next, we discuss weaning from the ventilator. Finally, we discuss some particular problems which are frequently asked about.

PHYSIOLOGIC BACKGROUND

A respirator needs to ensure adequacy of two specific functions: oxygenation and ventilation. Oxygenation refers, of course, to maintenance of a satisfactory arterial oxygen pressure (pO_2). Ventilation refers to maintenance of a satisfactory arterial carbon dioxide pressure (pCO_2).

One basic principle in the management of ventilators is that these two essential functions, oxygenation and ventilation, are separate and do not go hand in hand. This independence is brought out by considering how oxygenation and ventilation vary with changing minute volume (1). Minute volume is the product of respiratory rate and tidal volume. As can be seen from Fig. 1.1, **oxygenation is, in fact, independent of minute volume until ventilation falls very low**—so low that severe atelectasis occurs. House officers frequently fail to appreciate this phenomenon and increase

1

FIG. 1.1. Relationship of arterial pCO_2 and arterial O_2 saturation to minute volume. Note that pCO_2 varies inversely with minute volume and that O_2 saturation is largely independent of minute volume until minute volume falls very low. (Adapted from Ref. 1.)

minute volume in an ill-conceived attempt to improve oxygenation. On the other hand, **CO_2 removal is directly dependent on minute volume**. It is this relationship that renders the terms "CO_2 removal" and "ventilation" synonymous with regard to ventilator management.

Now what constitutes adequate oxygenation? Beginners often feel that pO_2 should be maintained at the normal level of 100 mm Hg that they are taught in physiology. In fact, of course, oxygenation is adequate at much lower pO_2 levels. What must be preserved is oxygen-carrying capacity per unit of blood. The well-known O_2–hemoglobin dissociation curve (Fig. 1.2) shows that at a pO_2 of 75 mm Hg blood is 95% saturated and at a pO_2 of 60 mm Hg blood is 90% saturated (2). Oxygen-carrying capacity is certainly well preserved at a pO_2 of 75 mm Hg and reasonably well preserved at a pO_2 of 60 mm Hg. So, **a pO_2 of 75 mm Hg is clearly adequate for all patients**, and a pO_2 of 60 mm Hg is probably adequate for all patients except those with severely limited blood flow to key organs (either from low cardiac output or from intrinsic vascular disease of the coronary arteries, extra-cranial cerebral vasculature, intestinal vasculature, or other specific vascular beds).

Next, what constitutes adequate ventilation? Here no leeway can be tolerated from the normal parameters familiar from physiology. In a patient on a ventilator, **pCO_2 should be strictly maintained at normal levels—that is, at 40 mm Hg or less**. Often we maintain pCO_2 in the 30–40 mm Hg range. There is probably no need to alter settings to increase a pCO_2 in the 30 mm Hg range. Many forces in critically ill patients tend toward acidosis. The patient may develop metabolic acidosis from hypoperfu-

FIG. 1.2. Oxyhemoglobin dissociation curve at 37°C and pH 7.4. (Adapted from Ref. 2.)

sion, hypovolemia, or sepsis. Respiratory acidosis may occur for many reasons: the endotracheal tube may dislodge or leak, the ventilator may malfunction or become disconnected, or a pneumothorax or major atelectasis may develop. In all such cases, a baseline mild respiratory alkalosis, which is well tolerated indefinitely, will have a protective effect against the forces toward acidosis. **Even in the face of total apnea, pCO_2 rises at about 3 mm Hg/min (3), so that maintenance of a mild respiratory alkalosis in ventilator patients may allow the critical several minutes required to remedy a malfunction** (to replace a dislodged endotracheal tube, for example).

Efficiency of ventilation is not commonly quantitated clinically, because ventilation is so efficient (by virtue of the greater ease of transport of CO_2 across the lung) that it suffers only in the preterminal stages of ventilatory dysfunction. Only very rarely is the house officer faced with critical impairment of CO_2 removal in patients on mechanical ventilation.

In severely ill patients, following both the **efficiency of oxygenation** and the adequacy of oxygenation may be required. The efficiency can be assessed by comparing the oxygen level provided in the alveolus to the oxygen level achieved in the blood. This parameter is quantitated as the $p(A - a)O_2$, the alveolar–arterial O_2 difference. This can be calculated by putting the patient on 100% oxygen and measuring the arterial pO_2. At 100% oxygen, the alveolus will contain only two other gases: water vapor at a partial pressure of 47 mm Hg and CO_2 at a partial pressure of 40 mm Hg (4). The sum of all partial pressures in the alveolus must equal atmospheric pressure (P_{atm}). Thus

$$p(A - a)O_2 = pAO_2 - paO_2$$
$$= (P_{atm} - pH_2O - pCO_2) - paO_2$$
$$= (760 - 47 - 40) - paO_2$$
$$= 673 - paO_2$$

where pAO_2 and paO_2 are alveolar and arterial O_2 pressures, respectively. A normal $p(A - a)O_2$ is 60–80 mm Hg (5). Thus in a normal patient on 100% O_2, arterial pO_2 levels of 600–620 mm Hg will be obtained. This is rarely realized in seriously ill ICU patients, in whom arterial pO_2 levels in the range of several hundred (on 100% O_2) are exceptionally good.

In patients with serious lung dysfunction, the $p(A - a)O_2$, if calculated on a daily basis, allows precise monitoring of the efficiency of oxygenation. Trends and consequences of treatment are noted sooner and are assessed more accurately if this parameter is followed.

PARAMETERS TO SET

When a patient is placed on a ventilator, as when returning to the ICU from the operating room, the following parameters need to be specified for the respiratory therapist to set up the machine:

Mode
Tidal volume
Respiratory rate
Fraction of inspired oxygen (FIO₂)
Positive end-expiratory pressure (PEEP)

It is presumed that a volume respirator is being set. Pressure ventilators, because of greater uncertainty in delivery of a satisfactory tidal volume, are no longer frequently used in intensive care settings, especially in surgical or cardiac ICUs.

Mode refers to the modality by which the ventilator will cycle. Until recent years, the available modes were mainly **controlled ventilation** and **assisted ventilation**. In controlled ventilation, the machine delivers a specified number of breaths per minute but does not allow the patient to breathe in between. In assisted ventilation, the machine senses the patient's inspiratory effort and delivers a breath at that time; in effect, it lets the patient decide when he needs a breath and then delivers that breath for the patient. Hybrids of these two modes are available as well.

In recent years the **intermittent mandatory ventilation (IMV)** mode has been introduced. In this mode, the machine delivers a specified number of breaths per minute at regular intervals but allows the patient to take a breath freely in between machine breaths. Despite common misconceptions, **there is not a patient in the hospital for whom IMV is not an appropriate mode of ventilation**. A very rare patient may be better served by one of the assist modalities (6), but even these patients can be very safely managed by appropriately set and adjusted IMV. The inexperienced house officer will still encounter respiratory therapists or nurses who object to

IMV on certain patients—preferring, for example, controlled ventilation for paralyzed patients and reserving IMV for patients capable of taking a breath. Those with this objection fail to realize that in this mode, as in controlled ventilation, the specified breaths will be delivered as reliably as in controlled ventilation. IMV need not be reserved for patients who can breathe and can capitalize on the feature of IMV that allows the patient to breathe freely between machine breaths.

Tidal volume refers, of course, to the volume of air to be cycled per machine breath. A normal tidal volume is approximately 5 ml/kg body weight, for spontaneous breathing. **For setting a ventilator, tidal volumes of 10–15 ml/kg are used.** This holds for newborns and infants as well as for adults. (For the very obese, nonobese body weight for frame size should be taken into account.) This 10–15 ml/kg represents an *initial* setting, to be modified based on arterial blood gas (ABG) determinations, as discussed in the next section.

Respiratory rate specifies the number of breaths per minute the machine is asked to deliver. **Rates of 8–12 are appropriate for adults;** 20–25 may be required for newborns; and 15–20 may be necessary for small children. These represent *initial* setting ranges at which these groups of patients are known to ventilate well; modifications, again, are based on ABG results.

FIO_2 refers to the fraction of oxygen in the delivered air. This can be expressed in percent (as in 28%, 50%, or 100% O_2) or in decimal form (as in 0.28, 0.50, or 1.00 O_2). **For initial settings after major surgery**, such as open-heart surgery or major abdominal, thoracic, or vascular procedures, **an initial FIO_2 of 1.0 is appropriate**. For lesser procedures, an initial FIO_2 of 0.5 should provide an adequate margin of safety for oxygenation. Again, initial settings will be modified based on ABG results.

PEEP refers to the amount of positive end-expiratory pressure to be maintained in the airways. Most experts feel that some physiologic PEEP is normally provided by an intact glottis. An endotracheal tube eliminates this normal physiologic mechanism responsible for keeping alveoli open. For this reason, most would agree that **every patient should be maintained on at least 5 cm H_2O of PEEP.**

ABG CONTINGENCIES AND PARAMETER RESETTING

The two functions the respirator must perform are oxygenation and ventilation. Adequacy of oxygenation is assessed entirely based on the arterial pO_2. Adequacy of ventilation is assessed entirely based on the arterial pCO_2. Thus, complex as ventilator management may seem to the beginner, all conceivable abnormalities of ventilator effectiveness can be grouped into four ABG contingencies (Fig. 1.3). These are the situations one must be prepared to handle:

pCO_2 may be too high.
pCO_2 may be too low.
pO_2 may be too high.
pO_2 may be too low.

If pCO_2 is too high, minute volume must be increased, either by increasing tidal volume or by increasing respiratory rate. As discussed earlier, pCO_2 varies inversely with minute volume, and increasing either tidal volume or respiratory rate will lower pCO_2. Now how does one choose which parameter to increase, tidal volume or respiratory rate? Here experience and judgment enter into the equation. If tidal volume is already at the upper limits of the suggested range, if peak inspiratory pressures are high, and if there is prominent chest expansion with each breath, one would be inclined to increase rate rather than volume. On the other hand, if the rate is already at the upper limits of the recommended range, if peak inspiratory pressures are low, and if chest expansion with each breath is not marked, tidal volume could safely and effectively be increased.

It should be noted that the adjustments described above presume that the pCO_2 is high despite proper functioning of the ventilator system. The pCO_2 may be high because the ventilator system is not delivering the prescribed minute volume. This may occur, for example, if there is a leak around the cuff of the endotracheal tube or in the ventilator tubing or connections, or if the endotracheal tube has been dislodged or was misplaced initially. When the pCO_2 is high, such problems must be checked for; it must be confirmed that the chest is moving and the breath sounds are good. The adjustments in tidal volume or respiratory rate are indicated once it is confirmed that the ventilator system is indeed delivering the minute volume initially set.

If the pCO_2 is too low, minute volume must be decreased, either by decreasing tidal volume or be decreasing respiratory rate. This is not a terribly serious condition, as it implies that one is ventilating the patient effectively—too effectively in fact. As discussed earlier, mild respiratory alkalosis is desirable. We would not ordinarily decrease minute volume unless the pCO_2 fell below 30 mm Hg. The decision about which parameter to decrease—tidal volume or respiratory rate—centers on the same considerations as earlier: Is the rate already relatively high? Is the volume already relatively high? How are the peak inspiratory pressures? How prominent is chest expansion?

| | | Modifications based on ABG contingencies | |
		pCO_2	pO_2
Initial settings:	High	↑ minute volume ↑ tidal volume ↑ respiratory rate	↓ FIO₂
Mode: IMV Tidal volume: 10-15 ml/kg Respiratory rate: 8-12/min FIO₂: 0.5 or 1.0 PEEP: 5 cm H₂O			
	Low	↓ minute volume ↓ tidal volume ↓ respiratory rate	PEEP ±↑ FIO₂ (if diffusion block)

FIG. 1.3. ABG contingencies in ventilator management. Appropriate initial respirator settings indicated on left. Diagram on right indicates appropriate modifications for ABG contingencies.

The issue of adjusting pCO_2 via dead space manipulation must be addressed. Some physicians will ask the therapist to add 6 or 12 inches of dead space to the ventilator tubing when the CO_2 is low. This seems to be done because of concern that lowering minute volume will adversely affect oxygenation. We have already established, however, that oxygenation is largely independent of ventilation. When this fact is appreciated, it becomes apparent that it is not necessary to use dead space to control pCO_2. Minute volume can be adjusted, and pO_2 will not suffer. In this way, certain dangers of dead space can be avoided. If a leak in the system should develop, the ventilation that is provided will not be wasted on an increased dead space. When the patient is weaned from the ventilator, he or she will not inadvertently be left breathing through an increased dead space. In our unit, dead space is *never* used to raise pCO_2.

What if pO_2 returns too high? This is not really a problem, as it signifies that the patient is oxygenating effectively—very effectively. **If the pO_2 is high—that is, above the 75 mm Hg we established as adequate—this provides the opportunity to lower FIO_2.** This is especially important if FIO_2 is above the potentially toxic levels of 0.5 or 0.6. If FIO_2 is below these levels and O_2 is still high, this is good, not bad; this implies efficient oxygenation. (We are not concerned here with the special matter of retrolental fibroplasia in newborns maintained at high blood pO_2.) No particular adjustment is required under these circumstances.

What if pO_2 returns too low? **If pO_2 is less than 75 mm Hg, especially if it is less than 60 mm Hg, serious hypoxia exists and remedial measures must be taken**. As will be made clear, increasing FIO_2 is usually not effective in postoperative patients; rather, **the treatment for hypoxia is PEEP** (7–10).

The overwhelming factor in postoperative hypoxia is atelectasis and its resultant ventilation–perfusion mismatch. Let us assume for illustrative purposes (Fig. 1.4) that we group all the ventilated alveoli in one lung and all the nonventilated alveoli in the other. If the patient is on 50% O_2 by endotracheal tube (Fig. 1.4A), conditions will be as follows. Blood entering either lung will be at mixed venous pO_2 and saturation levels—that is, at a pO_2 of 40 mm Hg and an O_2 saturation of 75%. Blood leaving the ventilated lung will be fully oxygenated in equilibrium with the alveolar pO_2, so that the effluent blood will have a pO_2 of about 300 mm Hg and an O_2 saturation in excess of 99%. Blood exiting the nonventilated lung will be unaltered, so that pO_2 will remain 40 mm Hg and saturation will be 75%.

Now if the patient is placed on 100% oxygen (Fig. 1.4B), conditions will be as follows. The blood flowing into either the ventilated or the nonventilated lung will have the same values as before—that is, the normal mixed venous values, pO_2 40 mm Hg and O_2 saturation of 75%. The blood leaving the ventilated lung will have a higher pO_2—say, 600 mm Hg—but the saturation will still be in excess of 99%. (This blood was already fully saturated on 50% inspired oxygen.) For the nonventilated lung, the effluent blood will still be fully desaturated; that is, pO_2 will be 40 mm Hg and O_2 saturation will be 75%. Thus increasing the inspired oxygen in the face of postoperative ventilation–perfusion mismatch will *not* appreciably improve oxygenation. This is because blood exiting ventilated alveoli is fully saturated already, and blood exiting nonventilated alveoli does not come in contact with the increased ambient oxygen.

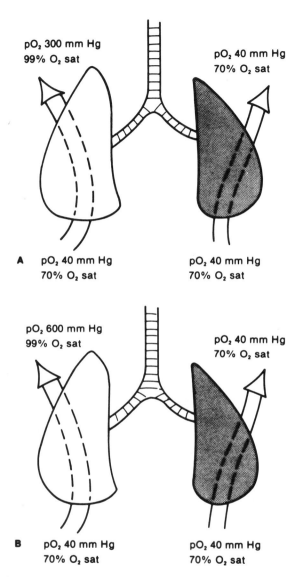

FIG. 1.4. Model for conceptualizing ineffectiveness of increasing inspired oxygen concentration to treat ventilation–perfusion mismatch. All ventilated alveoli are assumed to be concentrated in nonshaded lung and all nonventilated alveoli in shaded lung. (**A**) Conditions on 50% inspired oxygen; (**B**) conditions on 100% inspired oxygen.

FIG. 1.5. Arterial pO$_2$ as a function of shunt fraction (Q$_s$/Q$_t$) at different levels of FIO$_2$. (Reproduced with permission from Shoemaker WC, ed. *Textbook of critical care*. Philadelphia: WB Saunders; 1984.)

In this model, when blood from the two lungs mixes, half will be fully saturated and half will be fully unsaturated—just as before the FIO$_2$ was increased. (We have not considered here the amount of oxygen dissolved in plasma in addition to that bound to hemoglobin; this factor is negligible clinically.)

This very important principle regarding the ineffectiveness of increasing FIO$_2$ when there is ventilation–perfusion mismatch is confirmed graphically in Fig. 1.5, which plots resultant arterial pO$_2$ against shunt fraction. Shunt fraction represents that blood passing through unventilated alveoli. The severity of the shunt increases along the *x*-axis of the graph. The isobars represent different levels of alveolar O$_2$ (in mm Hg). As can be seen, even very high levels of inspired O$_2$ are ineffective in raising pO$_2$ when major shunting prevails.

To improve oxygenation, the nonventilated lung must be expanded; the ventilation–perfusion mismatch must be corrected. The key to accomplishing this is positive end-expiratory pressure, or PEEP, which alters the balance of forces toward preserving alveolar expansion. PEEP is usually begun at 5 cm H^2O. This is more or less a safe, physiologic level for all patients. PEEP can be added in increments of 2.5 or at most 5 cm H_2O (8,9). At times as much as 20, 25, or even 30 cm H_2O of PEEP may be required for a given patient. Most patients, however, are adequately handled by PEEP levels from 5 to 12.5 cm H_2O. Details concerning the dangers of PEEP will be covered later in this chapter.

In fairness, despite this emphasis on use of PEEP rather than increasing FIO_2 levels, there are certain settings in which it may be necessary to increase FIO_2 as well. This is the case, for example, where there is a block to diffusion of oxygen across the respiratory membrane, as in congestive heart failure and interstitial edema from adult respiratory distress syndrome. PEEP is effective in restoring ventilation–perfusion matching and may even alter the balance of forces away from interstitial edema, but it cannot overcome a severe diffusion block. In such a setting, it may be necessary to increase FIO_2 significantly.

WEANING FROM THE VENTILATOR

As is well appreciated, a patient must be surgically and hemodynamically stable in order to be safely weaned from the ventilator. Weaning and extubation are guided by: 1) ABGs and 2) respiratory mechanics. Most patients can be taken from IMV 8 to IMV 4 to "blow-by" (oxygen delivery only, without positive pressure ventilation) with ABGs being checked along the way. If pO_2 exceeds 75 mm Hg and pCO_2 is less than 45 mm Hg at each setting, weaning can proceed. It is important to maintain some positive end-expiratory pressure even when the patient is on blow-by. A usual PEEP level is 5 cm H_2O for this purpose. It is important not to leave a patient on blow-by for prolonged periods, usually no longer than 45 min, as the work of breathing is increased by the resistance to movement of air through the endotracheal tube. (Skeptics should try to breathe through a straw for a prolonged period.) If ABGs are acceptable at 45 min on blow-by with 5 cm H_2O positive airway pressure, this constitutes a satisfactory trial.

It is customary for the respiratory therapist to assess the respiratory mechanics during weaning or while the patient is on blow-by. The therapist will usually measure

Tidal volume
Vital capacity
Negative inspiratory force

during spontaneous ventilation. Tidal volume is often quite low and is not used as a criterion in our unit. If vital capacity is of the order of the tidal volume used during ventilation—that is, 10–15 ml/kg—mechanics are considered satisfactory for weaning or extubation. (This is much less than a normal vital capacity, of course.) A negative inspiratory force of -25 to -30 cm H_2O is considered satisfactory. It must be kept in mind that the mechanics recorded are highly dependent on patient understanding and cooperation for the exercise.

If ABGs and respiratory mechanics are satisfactory, extubation may safely be carried out. It must be recognized as well that although the beginner should not wean or extubate patients with unsatisfactory ABGs or mechanics, the experienced ICU physician often chooses to do so. Without this decision, certain patients might never satisfy weaning and extubation criteria. With careful judgment by experienced physicians, the vast majority of extubations under such circumstances are successful.

This chapter has covered how to set the ventilator initially, how to adjust respiratory parameters for the four categories of blood gas abnormalities, and how to withdraw mechanical ventilation, for essentially any patient in the hospital. What remains is to address special problems in respiratory management that are important for the neophyte.

SPECIAL PROBLEMS

Oxygen Toxicity

It is important to remember that **oxygen toxicity does not occur unless FIO_2 is maintained above 0.5 or 0.6 for more than 24 h (10)**. Thus placing the patient on 100% O_2 initially after returning from the operating room until a set of ABGs is obtained is not dangerous. Likewise, placing the patient on 100% O_2 for 20 min to calculate $p(A - a)O_2$ is not dangerous, and increasing FIO_2 briefly to treat an emergency is mandatory and *not* harmful. However, a patient left on 70% O_2 overnight unnecessarily after a coronary bypass will begin to accumulate significant periods of high O_2 ventilation. We make every attempt to get the FIO_2 to 0.5 or lower by using PEEP and by accepting a pO_2 of 75 mm Hg (or occasionally 60 mm Hg) as soon as possible after surgery. With this management outlook, if a particular patient should develop problems subsequently, he will not have accumulated time at dangerous FIO_2 levels.

PEEP Complications

PEEP is not without toxicity. A well-known toxic effect of PEEP is barotrauma— that is, the tendency for PEEP to increase peak inspiratory pressures and cause pneumothorax or pneumomediastinum. In a patient on positive pressure ventilation, of course, a pneumothorax from a parenchymal lung leak may expand rapidly and produce tension and hemodynamic compromise. Handling of this emergency is discussed in Chapter 16. The point to be emphasized here is that PEEP results in an increased end-expiratory lung volume and, consequently, decreased lung compliance. Thus the higher the PEEP level, the greater the increment in pressure associated with a given tidal volume.

Normal patients, when ventilated with tidal volumes in the range described, will have peak inspiratory pressures of 25–30 cm H_2O. The house officer should follow peak inspiratory pressure, which is displayed with each cycle by a gauge on the ventilator. Barotrauma does not occur when peak inspiratory pressure is less than 50 cm H_2O; barotrauma is seen in 8% of patients when peak pressure is 50–70 cm H_2O and in 43% of patients when peak pressure is greater than 70 cm H_2O (11). Most ventilators have a pop-off valve to prevent development of high pressures. The level for pop-off is set by the therapist, usually in the range of 60–70 cm H_2O. Above this pressure, an alarm sounds and the remaining tidal volume is vented and not delivered to the patient. Rarely, in critically ill patients with severe impairment of compliance, it may be necessary to disable or readjust the pop-off in order to ventilate the patient. In such a setting, the risk of pneumothorax must be accepted. The patient may even develop bilateral pneumothorax and have bilateral chest tubes placed in order to be ventilated adequately.

PEEP may have significant hemodynamic consequences as well (7–9). **Not only is the pressure of PEEP delivered into the bronchial tree, but some of the PEEP pressure is transmitted to the thorax and mediastinum**. Positive pressure in the thorax and mediastinum discourages filling of the right heart, and consequently of the left heart. By the Starling mechanism, stroke volume and cardiac output suffer. This is the basis for the well-known **depression of cardiac output by PEEP**. Blood pressure may fall and urine output may decrease. A patient with a normal heart may well tolerate 10 or 15 cm H_2O of PEEP without difficulty. Patients with sick hearts, especially postoperative cardiac patients, may tolerate PEEP very poorly. In a sick, postoperative mitral valve patient, 2.5 cm H_2O of PEEP may make the difference between a stable low-output state and frank cardiogenic shock.

The house officer should note as well that PEEP can artificially alter observed filling pressures. (See Chapter 5.)

Thus PEEP is useful and important, but dangerous. Its respiratory and hemodynamic consequences must constantly be kept in mind. Bear in mind also that positive pressure ventilation in and of itself, even without PEEP, has the same respiratory and hemodynamic consequences described earlier for PEEP, especially when peak inspiratory pressure is high. From this point of view, spontaneous ventilation, with the normally negative intrathoracic pressures, allows better cardiac filling and cardiac output than does positive pressure ventilation.

Mask O_2

The beginner often fails to realize that the designations of various face masks (40%, 60%, 100% mask) are **nominal** only. Many studies have demonstrated the limitations of such O_2 delivery systems (12–15). In fact, **it is impossible reliably to deliver greater than 50% O_2 except by endotracheal tube**. This has been determined by sampling tracheal O_2 in patients on various types of O_2 delivery apparatus. Nasal prongs have been shown to increase FIO_2 only insignificantly above room air levels. Even "100%" face masks do not deliver much more than 40% or 50% actual oxygen concentration. Face masks do not seal perfectly and in fact are designed so that the patient draws in air with each breath. If a normal inspiration lasts 1 second and involves movement of 500 ml of oxygen-enriched air, this represents an instantaneous flow of 30 liters/min. It would be impractical to supply flows of this magnitude for face masks. A corollary of these observations is that **one need not worry about O$_2$ toxicity in patients on a face mask**. (This regards actual O$_2$ toxicity to the lung. The well-known, though uncommon, suppression of hypoxic drive for ventilation in patients with chronic lung disease may occur with a face mask.)

Absorption Atelectasis

That increasing the FIO$_2$ may not improve oxygenation has already been explained. There is a way in which increasing the FIO$_2$ may actually impair oxygenation. When a patient is on 100% oxygen, there is no nitrogen in the alveolus. Nitrogen normally present in the alveolus, by virtue of its poor absorbability, provides some intra-alveolar positive partial pressure that acts as a so-called nitrogen stent for the alveolus (16). On 100% oxygen, or to a lesser extent on other high-oxygen concentrations, this nitrogen stent is lost or diminished. Atelectasis, called **absorption atelectasis** in this setting, may occur. Oxygenation may actually deteriorate. This is another factor in favor of using PEEP instead of raising FIO$_2$ to combat hypoxia.

Pressure Support Ventilation

A recent change in patterns of weaning patients from mechanical ventilation has been the advent of **pressure support ventilation** (PSV) (17), a new modality that has become popular with house officers and respiratory therapists and that has been incorporated into the setting menus of nearly all commercial ventilators. Traditional weaning patterns have been T-piece weaning (in which the patient is allowed to breathe completely without ventilator support for progressively longer periods of time) and IMV weaning (in which the number of breaths provided by the ventilator is progressively decreased). Both T-piece weaning and IMV weaning are often supplemented by conventional low-level positive end-expiratory pressure.

Pressure support ventilation is a new and different modality, in which, although the ventilator delivers no set mechanical breaths whatsoever, it senses the initiation of the patient's spontaneous breath and delivers a specified amount of pressure support during that breath. This support is like a "boost" or "tail wind" for the spontaneous breath, which makes the breath easier for the patient. The amount of pressure support can be varied over a continuous spectrum. High support corresponds to 15–18 cm H$_2$O and low support corresponds to to 5–8 cm H$_2$O. The pressure support increases the flow rate and the tidal volume significantly beyond what the native breath itself would achieve (Fig. 1.6). At high levels of pressure support, the work of breathing is nil and ventilation is fully supported mechanically. The house officer must remember, however, that unlike IMV, PSV does not deliver a single preprogrammed

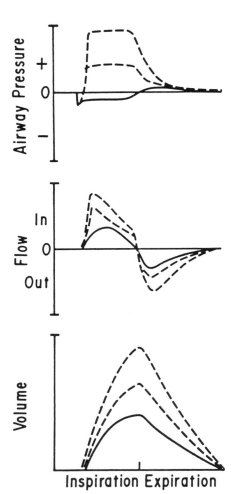

FIG. 1.6. Schematic representation of airway pressure (top panel), airflow (middle panel), and lung volume (lower panel). Solid lines depict a spontaneous breath without pressure support. Dotted lines depict two levels of pressure-support ventilation. Note higher airflow and larger volume of breath with pressure. Note also the patient's continued negative-pressure effort when unassisted, compared to the brief period of such patient effort when PSV is used. (Reproduced with permission from Ref. 17.)

breath, so an apneic patient, or one with inadequate respiratory drive, will not receive adequate ventilation. As the amount of PSV is decreased, the patient takes on more of the workload of breathing. At low levels of PSV, the positive pressure serves mainly to counteract the excess resistance of the endotracheal tube and ventilator as compared to the normal resistance without a tube.

Several paradigms for selection of initial setting of pressure level for high-level support in PSV have been proposed. One method is to apply one-third of the maximum inspiratory pressure observed during mechanical ventilation. (For example, the maximum inspiratory pressure for a given patient during conventional IMV ventilation is 45 cm H_2O; the initial pressure level selected for PSV is one-third of 45, or 15 cm H_2O.) Another method is to experiment with different levels of pressure support at the time of institution of PSV to determine and select that level of pressure support that yields a normal tidal volume for mechanical ventilation (i.e., 10–12 ml/kg).

Although most centers use PSV for specific weaning trials of finite duration, some maintain patients on PSV around the clock, gradually and progressively decreasing the amount of pressure support as the patient improves and strengthens.

Pressure support ventilation is intended for application not to the standard patient (e.g., the uncomplicated postcardiac surgical patient who is weaned quickly from the ventilator the morning after surgery), but to the more complicated or precarious patient who can be expected to require at least several days to wean from the ventilator. PSV is intended not for use while the patient is acutely ill, but for use later in recovery, when hemodynamics have stabilized and acute lung problems (atelectasis, edema, infiltrates) have cleared or improved. PSV clearly decreases the work of breathing. Patients respond very favorably, probably reflecting an improved coordination with the ventilator compared to IMV. In IMV, the prescribed breaths are interposed according to the machine's timing cycle. In PSV, the patient determines timing, depth, and frequency of breaths, with "boosting" of each breath by the pressure support. Dyspnea is minimized and patient comfort is dramatically improved. Nurses and allied personnel sense this feeling of improvement and respond favorably to PSV.

Although proponents argue for widespread application of PSV because of increased patient comfort and theoretical advantages, detractors point out that there is absolutely no clinical evidence that weaning is better or more effective with PSV (18) than with conventional modalities. Debate continues actively. Personal and institutional preferences abound. Progressively wider application of PSV appears likely, and the house officer must be familiar with the characteristics of this promising new modality of ventilation.

REFERENCES

1. West JB. *Pulmonary physiology—the essentials.* Baltimore: William & Wilkins; 1982.
2. George RB. Oxygen transport. In: George RB, Light RW, Matthay RA. eds. *Chest medicine.* New York: Churchill Livingstone; 1982:81–87.
3. Alfery DD, Benumof JL. Anesthesia for thoracic surgery. In: Miller RD, ed. *Anesthesia.* New York: Churchill Livingstone; 1981:925–980.
4. Guyton AC. Physical principles of gaseous exchange: diffusion of oxygen and carbon dioxide through the respiratory membrane. In: Guyton AC. *Textbook of medical physiology.* Philadelphia: WB Saunders; 1971:470–480.
5. Dunnill RPH, Crawley BB. *Clinical and resuscitative data.* Oxford: Blackwell; 1977.
6. Hudson LD. Intermittent mandatory ventilation (IMV). *Pulmonary Perspect* 1984;1:5–7.
7. Snyder JV, Carrol GC, Schuster DP, Culpepper J, Klain M. Mechanical ventilation: physiology and application. *Curr Probl Surg* 1984;2:1–87.
8. Shelhammer JH, Natason C, Parrillo JE. Positive end expiratory pressure in adults. *JAMA* 1984;251:2692–2695.
9. Luce JM. The cardiovascular effects of mechanical ventilation and positive end-expiratory pressure. *JAMA* 1984;252:807–811.
10. Winter PM, Miller NJ. Oxygen toxicity. In: Shoemaker W, Thompson W, Holbrook P, eds. *Textbook of critical care.* Philadelphia: WB Saunders; 1984:218–224.
11. Peterson GW, Baier H. Incidence of pulmonary barotrauma in a medical ICU. *Crit Care Med* 1983;11:67.
12. Shapiro BA, Harrison RA, Wolfson JR. *Clinical application of blood gases.* Chicago: Yearbook; 1977.
13. Gibson RL, Corner PB, Beckham RW, McGraw CP. Actual tracheal oxygen concentrations with commonly used oxygen equipment. *Anesthesiology* 1976;44:71–73.

14. Poulton TJ, Corner PB, Gibson RL. Tracheal oxygen concentrations with a nasal cannula during oral and nasal breathing. *Respir Care* 1980;25:739–741.
15. Schacter EN, Littner MR, Luddy P, Beck GJ. Monitoring of oxygen delivery systems in clinical practice. *Crit Care Med* 1980;8:405–409.
16. Vinocur B, Artz JS, Sampliner JE. Monitoring of respiratory status. In: Berk JL, Sampliner JR, Artz JS, Vinocur B, eds. *Handbook of critical care.* Boston: Little, Brown; 1976:57–86.
17. MacIntyre NR. Pressure support ventilation: effects on ventilatory reflexes and ventilatory-muscle workloads. *Respir Care* 1987;87:447–457.
18. Hughes CW, Popovich J Jr. Uses and abuses of pressure support ventilation. *J Crit Illness* 1989;4:25–32.

SUGGESTED FURTHER READING

Luce JM. The cardiovascular effects of mechanical ventilation and positive end-expiratory pressure. *JAMA* 1984;252:807–811.

An excellent review of the cardiovascular effects of PEEP including detailed discussion of effects on right and left ventricular function, the pulmonary vascular bed, cardiac output, and renal function.

MacIntyre NR. Pressure support ventilation: effects on ventilatory-muscle workloads. *Respir Care* 1987;32:447–457.

An excellent, unbiased presentation of the topic of PSV by one of its pioneers. The discussion of the paper serves to put the whole technique into perspective.

Schacter EN, Littner MR, Luddy P, Beck GJ. Monitoring of oxygen delivery systems in clinical practice. Crit Care Med 1980;8:405–409.

One of a number of experimental studies that make clear the lack of reliability of conventional prong and mask O2 delivery systems.

Snyder JV, Carrol GC, Schuster DP, Culpepper J, Klain M. Mechanical ventilation: physiology and application. *Curr Probl Surg* 1984;22:1–87.

A good review. Provides further details on many aspects of mechanical ventilation, including a section on high-frequency ventilation.

Winter PM, Miller, JN. Oxygen toxicity. In: Shoemaker W, Thompson W, Holbrook P, eds. *Textbook of critical care*. Philadelphia: WB Saunders; 1984:218–229.

An interesting review of basic research on oxygen toxicity, including a historical perspective and evidence on pathophysiology and treatment.

2 Arrhythmias

This chapter presents a simplified, fundamental approach to the management of acute alterations in cardiac rhythm. The perspective is primarily that of the care of the postoperative cardiothoracic patient, where many of the arrhythmias are most frequently seen. The principles are applicable as well in the coronary care unit and in the general surgical or medical intensive care unit.

The discussion is divided into three sections: bradycardias, supraventricular arrhythmias, and ventricular arrhythmias.

BRADYCARDIAS

The house officer should have a clearly organized armamentarium for the management of bradycardias, for these arrhythmias can be acutely life-threatening. The approach outlined here is valid for essentially all bradycardias, including sinus bradycardia, nodal bradycardia, and slow ventricular rhythm.

When does a bradycardia require treatment? Many patients exhibit slow rhythms but tolerate them well and do not require urgent intervention. Any thoracic ward, for example, frequently carries elderly patients whose pacemaker generators have failed. Most do not require any treatment other than semielective pacemaker generator replacement. Heart rate, of course, is a major determinant of cardiac output (output equals the product of heart rate and stroke volume). If cardiac output is maintained despite bradycardia, urgent treatment is not required. In the acute setting, adequacy of cardiac output is assessed by blood pressure and level of consciousness. If blood pressure is satisfactory, without dizziness, light-headedness, or disordered mentation, cardiac output is likely to be satisfactory. If these criteria are not met, cardiac output is unsatisfactory, and urgent treatment must be begun.

Even if blood pressure and consciousness are maintained, in most cases brady-cardia should be treated if the rate is below a certain absolute level. If the pulse is less than 45/min, and certainly if it is less than 40/min, treatment should be administered. Very few hearts, especially in the elderly or those with ischemic or valvular heart disease, can increase stroke volume enough to maintain cardiac output for sustained periods at pulse rates in this range. Also, with pulses this slow, dangerous ventricular foci may supervene.

There are three cardinal stages to the acute treatment of serious bradycardias (Fig. 2.1) (1)

1. **The initial treatment of choice is atropine.** This drug acts as a parasympatholytic agent to speed and encourage supraventricular, junctional, and ventricular foci and to promote atrioventricular (AV) conduction (2). Atropine is available as atropine sulfate in ampules containing 0.4 mg/ml or 0.5 mg/ml. The initial dose is 1 ml IV. An effect should be realized in 2–3 min. The dose should be repeated if no response is seen within this time. This drug is safe and should be used liberally. If no response is seen after the second dose, additional doses are unlikely to be effective, and one should move on to the second stage of treatment.

2. **If atropine is ineffective, the second drug of choice is isoproterenol (Isuprel).** If the parasympatholytic agent atropine is not effective, a β-agonist is required for its β-chronotropism. As is discussed in Chapter 7, Isuprel has a strong, almost pure β-activity. This makes it the next agent of choice in severe bradycardias. A convenient method of administration is by drip (2 mg/500 ml; again see Chapter 7). The drip is initially run quite fast (30, 60, or 120 ml/h or more, if required) until a pulse response is seen. The drug should be effective within minutes. It is important to slow the drip as soon as a pulse increment is observed, as untoward effects may be seen. Any patient can be thrown into ventricular fibrillation if Isuprel is infused fast enough. The infusion should be adjusted to achieve a safe rate, usually 60 ml/h or less.

3. **If Isuprel is ineffective, further pharmacologic efforts are futile, and emergency placement of a temporary cardiac pacemaker is indicated.** All physicians should know how to place temporary pacemakers. This is covered fully in Chapter 3.

It should be kept in mind that most postoperative cardiac patients have temporary pacemaker wires placed directly into the right ventricular myocardium and brought through the skin. These should be used, if available, when a postoperative cardiac patient requires temporary pacing.

SUPRAVENTRICULAR ARRHYTHMIAS

Supraventricular arrhythmias include sinus tachycardia, premature atrial contractions (PACs), atrial fibrillation, and atrial flutter (Fig. 2.2). Paroxysmal atrial tachycardia (PAT), seen commonly in healthy, young patients, is rarely encountered following

FIG. 2.1. Stepwise management of urgent bradyarrhythmias.

cardiac surgery. PAT and its variant MAT (multifocal atrial tachycardia) will not be specifically covered. When seen postoperatively, these rhythms can generally be approached as discussed later for atrial flutter.

Sinus tachycardia, PACs, atrial fibrillation, and atrial flutter in the postoperative cardiothoracic patient are all points on a spectrum of postoperative supraventricular irritability. Sinus tachycardia and frequent PACs often presage atrial fibrillation or flutter. A given patient may be in atrial fibrillation at one time and atrial flutter at another; over a period of days, the patient may convert back and forth from fibrillation or flutter to sinus rhythm, often with sinus tachycardia or PACs intervening.

Similar irritability can be seen in the coronary care unit with myocardial infarction or pericarditis; also, of course, these supraventricular arrhythmias can be seen in the coronary care unit in the setting of valvular heart disease or *de novo* without other primary structural heart disease.

In the case of noncardiac thoracic surgery, the more extensive the procedure, the greater the incidence of these supraventricular arrhythmias; that is, the incidence of arrhythmia is higher for pneumonectomy than for lobectomy, and higher for lobectomy than for simple exploration. Even in exploration without resection, however, there is a definite incidence of these arrhythmias. Though many causes have been postulated (direct irritation of the atrium, irritation of the pleura, disruption of parasympathetic atrial innervation), no clear explanation has been substantiated. It appears, however, that roughly one-half of patients undergoing pneumonectomies and one-third of patients undergoing lobectomies develop these arrhythmias.

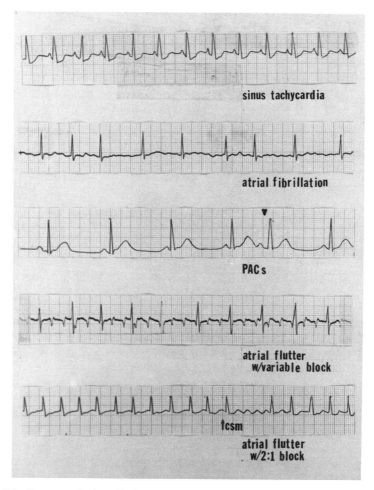

sinus tachycardia

atrial fibrillation

PACs

atrial flutter
w/variable block

↑csm

atrial flutter
w/2:1 block

FIG. 2.2. Supraventricular arrhythmias: illustrative EKGs. (csm, carotid sinus massage).

Much research has been directed into determining why supraventricular arrhythmias are seen so commonly after cardiac or thoracic surgery. Some have postulated that the venous cannula irritates the atrial pacemaking tissue. Withdrawal from rate-controlling antianginal medicines may be a factor in allowing tachycardias to develop. More recently, evidence suggests that conventional cardioplegia does not effectively quiet atrial activity, so that atrial pacemaking tissues may be rendered ischemic and irritable on that basis (3). In any case, at least a third of coronary bypass patients will develop these arrhythmias postoperatively. For patients with mitral valve dysfunction, supraventricular arrhythmias are part and parcel of the long-standing valvular heart disease with atrial enlargement. If the mitral patient has not already developed atrial fibrillation preoperatively, chances are that it will develop postoperatively.

Much effort has been directed toward developing methods to **prevent** these post-operative arrhythmias, but no clearcut solution has emerged. Prophylactic digitalization has yielded mixed results (4–6). Various protocols for resumption of β-blockers postoperatively appear promising (5,7). A recent meta-analysis (8), combining data from many studies on therapeutic strategies to prevent postoperative atrial fibrillation concluded that

1. Digitalis alone does not prevent post-operative atrial fibrillation.
2. β-blockers do discourage postoperative atrial fibrillation.
3. The combination of digitalis and β-blockers discourages postoperative atrial fibrillation more effectively than either drug administered alone.

Until more reliable prevention is available, these supraventricular arrhythmias will continue to be one of the cardiothoracic surgeon's most common problems.

Sinus Tachycardia

Sinus tachycardia usually has a physiologic cause; that is, the cardiovascular system attempts to compensate, to increase cardiac output, by increasing rate. The cause may be fever, pain, hypoxia, hypovolemia, low cardiac output, congestive heart failure, pulmonary embolus, or another primary disorder. The treatment for sinus tachycardia is that of the underlying physiologic disorder.

Fever and pain are especially common postoperative causes. Occasionally, however, a postoperative cardiac surgical patient will demonstrate sinus tachycardia, although he or she is well in all other respects: The patient is not febrile and has no severe pain; vital signs, physical examination, and urine output suggest good cardiac output; hematocrit is stable; and chest x-ray and electrocardiogram are satisfactory. The cause for tachycardia in this setting is not at all clear. Some believe that withdrawal of β-blockers and calcium antagonists (given preoperatively for angina) may be responsible. In any case, in this setting, when the patient has sinus tachycardia and all investigations fail to disclose any physiologic abnormality, it is permissible to treat the tachycardia with β-blockers. Usually, 10 or 20 mg of propranolol (Inderal) orally four times daily will suffice. Metoprolol (Lopressor) 25–50 mg orally twice daily is also effective. Often this medication can be discontinued after several weeks without recurrence of tachycardia.

Premature Atrial Contractions

PACs in themselves are not dangerous. They are supraventricular beats conducted along standard pathways from the AV node downward, so they produce a coordinated ventricular contraction. Usually, unless they occur very early in the cardiac cycle, PACs produce an effective pressure pulse and thus do not adversely affect cardiac output. Unlike PVCs, they do not presage life-threatening ventricular arrhythmias. However, as indicated, **frequent PACs, especially after cardiac or thoracic**

surgery, portend impending atrial fibrillation; this requires prophylactic digitalization. The purpose of digitalization in this setting is to control the rate of ventricular response should atrial fibrillation supervene.

Atrial Fibrillation

When a young, healthy patient develops atrial fibrillation, the rate of ventricular response can be quite rapid, at times as high as 180/min or 200/min (4). In the elderly, sick patient, ventricular response is usually on the order of 140–160/min. Although a young, healthy heart may be able to maintain cardiac output at rates in this range, most hospitalized and postoperative patients cannot compensate. Tachycardia occurs at the expense of diastole. Stroke volume is decreased because filling time is short. In addition, increased heart rate leads to increased myocardial oxygen demand, and the shortened diastolic time results in decreased coronary flow and hence decreased oxygen supply. This alteration in myocardial oxygen supply and demand results in myocardial ischemia, with its negative inotropic effect also contributing to decrease the stroke volume. Atrial fibrillation with a rapid response represents a serious insult to the patient's physiology. **The goal in acute management is not to restore sinus rhythm** (which, even if achieved, cannot usually be maintained) **but to effect control of rate.**

We have found it useful to separate patients with new-onset atrial fibrillation into three categories of urgency (Table 2.1).

Level I (Relatively Nonurgent)

A postoperative coronary bypass patient goes into atrial fibrillation on postoperative day 1. His rate is 145/min; blood pressure is 120/80 mm Hg. He is awake, alert, and responds appropriately to questions. He has no chest pain.

Table 2.1 *Treatment of atrial fibrillation by level of urgency*

Urgency level	Signs	Treatment
Level I	Pulse: 120-140/min BP: >100 mm Hg Satisfactory level of conciousness No angina	Digitalis
Level II	Pulse: 140-160/min BP: 80-100 mm Hg Possible dizziness Possible mild angina	Digitalis plus Inderal/verapamil
Level III	Pulse: 140-160+/min BP: <80 mm Hg Impaired level of conciousness Angina	DC cardioversion

This patient falls into the first, lowest category of urgency. Treatment for this patient is rapid digitalization. **Digitalis is the only available drug that slows ventricular response without adversely affecting myocardial contractility**. Several schemes of administration can be used. One rule of thumb is that digoxin, 0.9 mg/m² of body surface area, given intravenously in divided doses over 24 h, will effect satisfactory digitalization. For practical purposes, for the average-sized adult, 0.5 mg IV initially and 0.25 mg IV every 6 h for two or three additional doses (a total digitalizing dose of 1.0–1.25 mg) will usually digitalize adequately without overdosing. Subsequently, a daily maintenance dose, usually 0.25 mg IV or p.o., can be started.

A particular patient may not slow with the initial 0.5-mg IV dose. Here the pharmacokinetics of intravenous digitalis come to bear. Onset of action for intravenous digoxin takes as long as 30 min; peak effect may not occur for 90–120 min (9). Thus one should not expect an immediate or rapid effect. Likewise, **digoxin doses should not in general be given at intervals of less than 2 h**; otherwise the full effect of previous doses may not be realized and toxicity from additive effect may be induced.

A very important point is that **digoxin levels have little bearing on the acute management of new-onset atrial fibrillation. The best indicator of adequacy of digitalization is the rate of ventricular response in atrial fibrillation. Digitalis can be administered with impunity** (with the preceding caveats as to dosage intervals) **until the rate is controlled to 120/min or less** (1). Digoxin levels are not routinely available on an emergency basis. The levels are always tremendously high when drawn shortly after intravenous doses.

Thus if a particular patient does not slow after the initial digoxin dose, additional drug may be given, usually 0.25 mg IV, every 2 h until the heart rate slows. The rate should be slowed at least to 120/min. Often we will slow the response to 90–100/min to optimize ventricular filling between beats and lower myocardial oxygen demands.

This paradigm presumes that the rhythm is indeed atrial fibrillation. The impunity in dosage does not hold for other rhythms. Also, some reasonable maximum limit must be put on the amount of digitalis administered. In our unit no more than 2.5 mg of digoxin is administered in one 24-h period.

Level II (Somewhat Urgent).

A postoperative coronary bypass patient goes into atrial fibrillation on postoperative day 1. Heart rate is 160/min; blood pressure is 90/50 mm Hg. The patient is awake but somewhat confused. He feels some mild chest discomfort coming on.

This patient is clearly in more jeopardy than the one described earlier. He qualifies for our second level of urgency. As for the first patient, digitalis will be the key to control of ventricular response for this patient. Digitalis should be given immediately, as previously. However, this patient cannot wait the 30 min it may take for digitalis to act. His rate needs to be slowed quickly. **Two categories of drugs are available for intravenous use that can slow the ventricular response within minutes: β-blockers and calcium antagonists.** The β-blocker of choice has been propranolol

(Inderal), and the calcium antagonist of choice has been verapamil (Calan). Both categories of agents can be used effectively.

Inderal can be counted on to slow the rate reliably and in gradual fashion. It is important to realize that the intravenous dose of Inderal is much smaller than the oral dose, with a rough equivalency of 1 mg IV to 10 mg p.o. Errors have been made, with junior house officers giving an oral dose intravenously. Inderal is administered as 1 mg IV push every 3–5 min until the desired slowing of rate is achieved. (In the very early hours after surgery, it may be best to start with 0.25 or 0.5 mg). Up to 10 mg can be given at intervals in one session. Administration should be stopped when the rate reaches 120/min or less. Again, the goal is not to restore sinus rhythm but to control the ventricular response.

Verapamil can also be used effectively (10). The effect from verapamil may be more dramatic—a sudden slowing of rate or, at times, a conversion to sinus rhythm— but less controlled than that of Inderal. Verapamil may be given as 5 mg IV over several minutes, with the dose repeated every 10–15 min to a total of 15 mg at one sitting.

Important points to remember are the following:

- Both categories of agent can cause bradycardia and heart block. If the patient is a postoperative open-heart patient, the pacing wires should be connected to an external pacemaker set on the stand-by mode. If no pacing wires are available, measures should be taken to ensure that the drugs and equipment necessary for treating bradycardias (see earlier) are available.
- **Intravenous β-blockers and calcium antagonists are not ordinarily used together, for their combined negative chronotropic and inotropic effects can be overwhelming in certain patients** (11). **Asystole may occur** (11,12). In our unit, if intravenous β-blockers are chosen initially, intravenous calcium antagonists are not used for 4 h, and vice versa. The experienced physician may make exceptions to this rule in selected cases.
- The use of β-blockers and calcium antagonists described earlier is crisis intervention. Once the rate is slowed or conversion to sinus rhythm is attained, the life-threatening condition is averted. However, when the β-blocker or calcium antagonist effect wears off, the arrhythmia is likely to recur, because the propensity for rapid rate is still present. This is why concurrent digitalization is imperative. Beginning an oral dose of β-blocker (often Inderal 10–20 mg p.o. q6h) or calcium antagonist (usually 80 mg verapamil p.o. q8h) can help to maintain sinus rhythm and to assure a controlled rate if atrial fibrillation recurs. Various new long-acting B-blockers and calcium antagonists are now available that allow the convenience of once- or twice-a-day dosing. (See Chapter 21.)

Level III (Urgent).

A postoperative coronary bypass patient goes into atrial fibrillation on postoperative day 1. His heart rate is 180/min. He loses consciousness and his blood pressure falls to 60 mm Hg systolic. Just before losing consciousness, he complained of chest pain and clutched his chest.

This patient is acutely threatened. He is in a higher category of urgency than either of the two patients described thus far. **The treatment for rapid atrial fibrillation with severe compromise of vital signs is direct current (DC) cardioversion.** Details regarding use of the defibrillator are reviewed in Chapter 4. Atrial fibrillation usually responds quite well, with return of normal sinus rhythm at a controlled rate. Following cardioversion, intravenous digitalization is in order, because the arrhythmia is likely to reappear. Oral maintenance Inderal (or other β-blocker) or verapamil (or other calcium antagonist) may also be instituted for further suppression and rate control.

In recent years, multiple new intravenous drugs have become available for the control of the ventricular response in atrial fibrillation, including both β-blockers and calcium antagonists. (See Table 2.2.)

Esmolol (13) is a very useful short-acting, cardioselective β-blocker for IV administration. It has a quick onset of action and a similarly short duration of action after discontinuation (half-life 9 min). The calcium antagonist diltiazem is available in intravenous form for both bolus and continuous infusion. Diltiazem has a long duration of action (half-life 3.4 h). Titration of infusion rate to therapeutic effect is key with both esmolol and diltiazem. Care should be exercised in administration to patients with underlying hemodynamic compromise not directly related to rapid ventricular response. Choice among the agents listed in Table 2.2 is largely based on individual or institutional preference. The use of IV bolus or continuous infusion agents is limited to the period of time required for oral treatment with β-blockers or calcium antagonists to take effect.

Atrial Flutter

Atrial flutter represents another point on the spectrum of supraventricular arrhythmias. A given patient may have PACs at one moment, fibrillation at another, and flutter at still another. The atrial rate in flutter is about 300/min. Fortunately, conduction is usually 2:1 or less; that is, only one-half or fewer of the impulses reaching the AV node are conducted to the ventricle.

Table 2.2. *Drugs for IV administration for the control of ventricular response in atrial fibrillation.*

	β-Blockers			Calcium antagonists	
	IV bolus (over 3 min.)	IV infusion		IV bolus (over 3 min.)	IV infusion
Propranolol (Inderal)	1mg (up to 10 mg)	NA	**Verapamil** (Isoptin)	2.5-5 mg	NA
Esmolol (Brevibloc)	0.5 mg/kg	0.05-0.2 mg/kg/min	**Diltiazem** (Cardizem)	0.25 mg/kg	5-15 mg/h

The treatment of atrial flutter closely parallels that of atrial fibrillation. The objective, as with fibrillation, is control of rate rather than restoration of sinus rhythm. The same categories of treatment for the same general levels of urgency apply.

The following points regarding atrial flutter should be kept in mind:

- **Flutter is underdiagnosed by the house officer**. Especially in a postoperative open-heart patient, a perfectly regular rhythm with a ventricular response of 150/min is flutter with 2:1 block much more often than not. Flutter waves may not be seen at 2:1 conduction; carotid sinus massage to increase block even transiently to 3:1 conduction will clearly show flutter waves (see Fig. 2.2). With 2:1 conduction, this rhythm is often mistaken for sinus or PAT. Of note as a distinguishing feature is the paroxysmal nature of flutter as opposed to sinus tachycardia. If the rate jumps suddenly to 150/min, that argues for flutter and against sinus tachycardia.
- In atrial flutter, unlike in atrial fibrillation, digitalization cannot be guided with impunity by the ventricular rate. Although the ventricular response gradually decreases with digitalization in atrial fibrillation, atrial flutter may be resistant to digitalis, and a sudden increase in block may occur, or another manifestation of digitalis toxicity may be seen (1). If block changes from 2:1 to 3:1 initially, and then suddenly with more digitalis to, say, 10:1, the ventricular response will only be 30/min. It is best with flutter to give just a calculated appropriate total dose of digitalis in divided doses and then to use other agents. Here digoxin levels may be helpful on subsequent days.
- **Atrial flutter is exquisitely sensitive to cardioversion**. Usually 10 joules suffices to convert to normal sinus rhythm.
- **Atrial flutter may at times be treated very effectively with overdrive pacing** (14). At centers where house staff are familiar with this technique, conversion to normal sinus rhythm may be accomplished quickly and easily. (Again, see Chapter 3 for details.) Even if overdrive pacing is used, digoxin with or without β-blockers or calcium antagonists should be begun for easier rate control when the flutter recurs.

On subsequent days, after the acute problems of new-onset fibrillation or flutter have been controlled, some physicians may choose to add quinidine or procainamide (Pronestyl) to help maintain sinus rhythm and discourage recurrence of the arrhythmia. Quinidine may be started at 300 mg p.o. q6h and Pronestyl at 375 mg p.o. q4h. A newer, longer-acting, sustained-release form of Pronestyl (Procan-SR) may be given every 6 h, usually at 500 mg p.o. Therapy is guided by serum levels of these two drugs. These agents are not useful in the acute management of new-onset atrial fibrillation or flutter; in fact, they are usually contraindicated because they promote AV conduction and may **increase** the rate of ventricular response. These agents can safely be used only if complete digitalization has been achieved.

Recent studies have shown that both quinidine and procainamide may have serious deleterious effects, especially a pro-arrhythmic effect in up to 15% of treated patients. In these patients, serious ventricular arrhythmias may be seen, as a consequence of the prolongation of the QT interval by these drugs. **Specifically, the**

particular arrhythmia known as *torsades de pointe*, deriving its French name from the undulation of the electrogram away from and then close to the baseline, **is a serious variant of ventricular tachycardia seen from quinidine or procainamide toxicity** (Fig. 2.3).

When quinidine or procainamide is begun, drug levels must be monitored closely if toxicity is to be avoided. In addition, the QT interval must be followed carefully, often daily. A prolongation in the QT interval often precedes pro-arrhythmic toxicity. The QT interval is measured from the beginning of the QRS complex to the end of the T wave. The QT interval must be adjusted for heart rate, as the interval normally decreases with increasing heart rate. The QT_c, or corrected QT interval, is calculated by dividing the QT by the square root of the R-R interval. (Many contemporary automated EKG machines print out the QT and QT_c directly.) **A QT_c of greater than 400 msec should raise concern over the potential for proarrhythmic toxicity.**

There has been a high level of interest among house officers recently in the antiarrhythmic agent adenosine. Adenosine (the naturally occurring nucleotide in intravenous form) is unique in that it is metabolized in seconds (half-life less than 10 seconds). **Adenosine causes very transient interruption of conduction through the A-V node.** This interruption lasts only seconds, so it is virtually impossible to cause any lasting harm by administration of this drug. Contrary to a burgeoning reputation that this drug is a panacea for all manner of supraventricular arrhythmias, in fact, adenosine is useful therapeutically only for paroxysmal supraventricular tachycardia (PSVT). This abruptly occurring rhythm is often seen in young patients without structural heart disease. This is a reentrant tachycardia that depends on a circular conduction of impulses through two pathways between the atrium and ventricle. Wolff-Parkinson-White syndrome patients, and others, can develop such reentrant supraventricular tachycardias. By virtue of interruption of the A-V node limb of the reentrant circuit, adenosine is extremely effective at terminating PSVT and restoring sinus rhythm. The dose is 6 or 12 mg given by IV bolus. Despite misconceptions to the contrary, aside from a transient slowing of ventricular response, atrial fibrillation and atrial flutter are not impacted in any lasting fashion by administration of adenosine. Although this transient increase in degree of block, may, like carotid sinus massage, make the fibrillation or flutter easier to recognize on EKG, there is no direct therapeutic benefit.

FIG. 2.3. Torsades de pointe.

It should be kept in mind that, by one or two months after open-heart surgery, except in patients with long-standing arrhythmias or valvular heart disease, the postoperative supraventricular irritability disappears. β-blockers, calcium antagonists, antiarrhythmics, and even digitalis can usually be discontinued at this point.

VENTRICULAR ARRHYTHMIAS

The discussion of ventricular arrhythmias will be divided into three sections: premature ventricular contractions (PVCs), ventricular tachycardia, and ventricular fibrillation (Fig. 2.4).

Premature Ventricular Contractions

Ventricular ectopic beats are threatening in two ways: They impair cardiac output, and they presage more serious ventricular arrhythmias. Unlike PACs, PVCs do not originate supraventricularly and do not propagate along specialized conducting tissues. For this reason, the cardiac contraction with a PVC is less "coordinated" than

FIG. 2.4. Ventricular arrhythmias: illustrative EKGs.

with a supraventricular beat. This can usually be seen in the arterial trace as a drop in arterial pressure, or a total lack of pressure spike, for the ectopic beat. As is well known, PVCs may be the forerunner of ventricular tachycardia or ventricular fibrillation.

In the postoperative coronary patient, as in the patient with acute myocardial infarction, the general irritability of the heart argues for aggressive treatment of PVCs. If the PVCs are frequent (more than 6/min), multifocal (manifested by multiple EKG configurations), or occurring in couplets or runs, treatment should be undertaken.

The first-line drug for ventricular ectopy is lidocaine. The initial dose is 1 mg/kg (given by IV push). This is usually followed by a continuous infusion at 1–4 mg/min. An additional bolus of 0.5 mg/kg can be administered, along with an increase in the drip rate, if the initial bolus and drip do not control the arrhythmia (15). **Lidocaine does cause CNS effects (especially seizures) in high doses**; administration at 4 mg/min should not be maintained any longer than absolutely necessary. Lidocaine is a very effective drug. Control of the PVCs is usually seen within 1 or 2 min. If lidocaine does not control the arrhythmia, chances are that other agents will not. However, Pronestyl can be tried. The loading dose is 100 mg for every 10 kg of body weight. Each 100 mg must be given over 5–10 min. **Pronestyl is a potent negative inotropic agent** and may drop blood pressure, especially in sensitive postoperative cardiac patients. The house officer should watch for QRS widening, which may indicate impending toxicity. The loading dose can be followed by a drip, as for lidocaine, at 1–4 mg/min.

If neither lidocaine nor Pronestyl is effective, chances are the ectopy will not respond to drugs. However, bretylium is occasionally effective in refractory ventricular arrhythmias of this sort. Occasionally, some patients in our unit respond dramatically to bretylium and to bretylium only. The initial dose is 5 mg/kg by IV push. This can be repeated if required for control. The initial dose may be followed by a continuous infusion of 1–2 mg/min. **Bretylium is a potent peripheral vasodilator**; volume expanders, inotropes, and vasoconstrictors should be available during institution of therapy to combat the vasodilation if required.

Ventricular Tachycardia

Ventricular tachycardia refers to a rapid, usually regular, wide-complex rhythm of ventricular origin. House officers often fail to appreciate that **ventricular rhythms may at times sustain good hemodynamics**. Although each contraction is not as coordinated as a normally conducted beat, it may produce a satisfactory stroke volume. After all, ventricular pacing, which is so commonly instituted for maintenance of cardiac output in patients with bradycardia or heart block, produces essentially a ventricular rhythm.

If hemodynamics are maintained by the ventricular rhythm, the treatment of choice is lidocaine, followed by Pronestyl or bretylium if required. Particulars of administration are the same as for PVCs.

If hemodynamics are not sustained in ventricular tachycardia, the treatment of choice is electrical conversion. Details regarding the use of the defibrillator are covered in Chapter 4.

Ventricular Fibrillation

Ventricular fibrillation, with its chaotic, constant myocardial contractions, **can never sustain hemodynamics. The treatment for ventricular fibrillation is immediate defibrillation**. Again, see Chapter 4 for details.

The early postoperative period after cardiac surgery and the period following an acute myocardial infarction represent times of severe ventricular irritability. The operated heart has been handled, incised, cannulated, cooled, warmed, and sutured. It is far from surprising that it is irritable. Also, the postoperative period is one of electrolyte flux. Polyuria after bypass can exceed 1 liter/h. Forty or 60 mEq of potassium may be lost with each liter, sometimes within 1 h. For all these reasons, ventricular fibrillation may develop after cardiac surgery even in patients who are otherwise perfectly well. The arrhythmia must be detected immediately, recognized immediately, and treated immediately by defibrillation. On any cardiac service, in the course of one year, at least several patients will have fibrillated, been defibrillated immediately, and recovered without problem, being discharged at the usual time. The key here is immediate recognition by the house officer, followed by defibrillation; hesitation may result in mortality.

General Approach to Arrhythmias

There are several questions that house officers must ask themselves in evaluating any arrhythmia:

1. **What is the rhythm**? This question is of obvious importance.
2. **Is it hurting the patient?** Different arrhythmias cause different degrees of physiologic disturbance. Some need urgent treatment (as in rapid atrial fibrillation with alteration in vital signs, or in ventricular fibrillation). Others may require no additional treatment at all (as in recurrence of atrial fibrillation with a controlled rate in an already digitalized patient).
3. **What is causing the arrhythmia?** House officers are usually quite thorough in investigating factors that may be responsible for arrhythmias. These include the following:
   a. **Electrolytes**. Potassium is especially critical. In settings of ventricular irritability or digitalis administration, serum potassium should be maintained at 4.5 mEq/liter or greater. Sodium also may be important. Calcium and magnesium levels may be investigated.
   b. **ABGs.** Hypoxia certainly can cause arrhythmias, as can acidosis.
   c. **EKG.** A 12-lead EKG must be evaluated for evidence of ischemia as the factor causing the arrhythmia

d. **The Swan-Ganz Catheter**. One factor that is often overlooked is the Swan-Ganz catheter. The tip of this catheter can drop back through the pulmonary valve into the right ventricle and irritate the myocardium, causing ventricular ectopy. A loop of catheter also may cause ectopy if it rubs on the ventricular wall. This must constantly be kept in mind, especially when ectopy is unexpected from the patient's general physiologic condition and when ectopy occurs in runs of PVCs with entirely normal intervening periods. In this setting, the ectopy may be accompanied by a change in the Swan-Ganz trace from that typical of pulmonary artery placement to a right ventricular configuration. The catheter must be withdrawn out of the heart into a central venous position if it is thought to be the cause of life-threatening ectopy. (See Chapter 5 for further discussion of Swan-Ganz catheter positioning.)

4. **Is digitalis involved?** Digitalis excess can cause essentially any arrhythmia. In our ICU, we review in detail the complete "digitalis history" whenever an arrhythmia occurs. This involves ascertaining exactly how much digitalis was given when—including preoperatively, intraoperatively, and postoperatively. Digitalis levels may help as well.

5. **How do I treat it?** Only after the preceding questions are asked and answered can a treatment plan be formulated appropriately. The preceding discussion covers particular treatment of specific arrhythmias.

By rigorously asking these questions in all cases, the house officer can be assured of not overlooking significant data points. By gathering data in this way and applying the principles outlined for specific arrhythmias, one can be assured of providing appropriate care for acute disturbances of cardiac rhythm.

REFERENCES

1. Kirklin J, Daggett WM, Lappas DG. Postoperative care following cardiac surgery. In: Johnson RA, Haber E, Austen WG, eds. *The practice of cardiology.* Boston: Little, Brown; 1980:1110–1132.
2. Innes IR, Nickerson M. Drugs inhibiting the action of acetylcholine on structures innervated by postganglionic parasympathetic nerves (antimuscarinic or atropinic drugs). In: Goodman LS, Gilman A, eds. *The pharmacologic basis of therapeutics.* New York: Macmillan; 1970.
3. Smith PK, Buhrman WC, Levett JM, et al. Supraventricular conduction abnormalities following cardiac operations: a complication of inadequate atrial preservation. *J Thorac Cardiovasc Surg* 1983;85:105–115.
4. Tyras DH, Stothert SC Jr, Kaiser GC, et al. Supraventricular tachyarrhythmias after myocardial revascularization: a randomized trial of prophylactic digitalization. *J Thorac Cardiovasc Surg* 1979;77:310–314.
5. Roffman JA, Fieldman A. Digoxin and propranolol in the prophylaxis of supraventricular tachydysrhythmias after coronary artery bypass surgery. *Ann Thorac Surg* 1980;31:496–501.
6. Csicsko JF, Schatzlein MH, King PD. Immediate postoperative digitalization in the prophylaxis of supraventricular arrhythmias following coronary artery bypass. *J Thorac Cardiovasc Surg* 1981;81:419–422.
7. Mohr R, Smolinsky A, Goor DA. Prevention of supraventricular tachyarrhythmia with low-dose propranolol after coronary bypass. *J Thorac Cardiovasc Surg* 1981;81:840–845.
8. Kowey PR, Taylor JE, Rials SJ, Merinchak RA. Meta-analysis of the effectiveness of prophylactic drug therapy in preventing supraventricular arrhythmia early after coronary bypass grafting. *Am J Cardiol* 1982;69:963–965.

9. Moe GK, Farah AE. Digitalis and allied cardiac glycosides. In: Goodman LS, Gilman A, eds. *The pharmacologic basis of therapeutics*. New York: Macmillan; 1970.
10. Plumb VJ, Karp RB, Kouchoukos NT, et al. Verapamil therapy of atrial fibrillation and atrial flutter following cardiac operation. *J Thorac Cardiovasc Surg* 1982;83:590–596.
11. Urthaler F, James JN. Experimental studies on the pathogenesis of asystole after verapamil in the dog. *Am J Cardiol* 1979;44:651–656.
12. Benarm MD Asystole after verapamil. *Br Med J* 1972;2:169–170.
13. Shettigar UR, Toole JG, Appunn DO. Combined use of esmolol and digoxin in the acute treatment of atrial fibrillation or flutter. *Am Heart J* 1993;126:368–374.
14. Waldo AL, MacLean WAH, Karp RB, et al. Entrainment and interruption of atrial flutter with atrial pacing: studies in man following open heart surgery. *Circulation* 1977;56:737–745.
15. Lewis, ed. *Textbook of advanced cardiac life support*. Dallas: American Heart Association; 1981:VIII-1–VIII-16.

SUGGESTED FURTHER READING

Benarm MD. Asystole after verapamil. *Br Med J* 1972;2:169–170.
Urthaler F, James JN. Experimental studies in the pathogenesis of asystole after verapamil in the dog. *Am J Cardiol* 1979;44:651–656.

These two articles will serve to give the house officer a healthy respect for the dangers of combining β-blockers and verapamil.

3 Temporary Pacemakers

The postoperative cardiac patient, the patient with coronary ischemia, and the post-myocardial infarction patient are all at risk for bradycardia. Regarding the postoperative cardiac patient, the cooling associated with cardiopulmonary bypass, the cardioplegia, and the ischemia during the cross-clamp period all may affect the pace-making tissues and conducting system of the heart. Patients who have had valve surgery may have operative injury to, or edema of, the His bundle, which can lead to sudden heart block. Further, hypotension of any cause in the postoperative period may lead to hypoperfusion of the heart and cause bradycardia.

Thus the house officer who cares for acutely ill patients must be prepared to treat a sudden bradycardia at any time. The general management of bradycardia has been covered in Chapter 2. The postoperative cardiac patient almost always has temporary epicardial pacing wires placed specifically to allow reliable pacing in case of post-operative bradycardia. This chapter will concentrate on the basics of pacing with these wires and with other temporary systems and on the use of the temporary external pacemakers themselves.

OPERATIVE PLACEMENT OF PACING WIRES

The epicardial wires placed at the time of cardiac surgery are insulated except at the tip near the curved needle (Fig. 3.1). The curved needle is used to pass the wire through the myocardium. The ventricular wire is usually placed in the anterior wall of the right ventricle at a spot free of fat where the myocardium shows clearly (Fig. 3.2). The curved needle is then cut off, the wire is positioned so that the uninsulated portion is in touch with the heart muscle, and it is secured. The end with the straight needle is passed through the body wall and the wire is secured to the skin to prevent dislodgement. The sharp tip is cut off, and the remaining portion of the straight nee-

33

FIG. 3.1. Epicardial pacing wire.

dle serves as a contact. At the time of discharge, the wire can be easily pulled out by gentle traction. A separate ground wire is placed in the skin only (with the curved needle end). Again, care is taken that the uninsulated portion is actually in touch with the skin.

Atrial pacing wires are placed somewhat differently. Because of the thin atrial wall, the wire is not passed through but is affixed to the atrial surface by suture.

When not in use, the external contacts of the pacing wires should be insulated from external electrical forces. This can be done by securing the needles between two pieces of tape or by putting them into a test tube or plastic needle sheath. Without this precaution an electrical short circuit from bedside electrical equipment could conceivably be conducted to the heart.

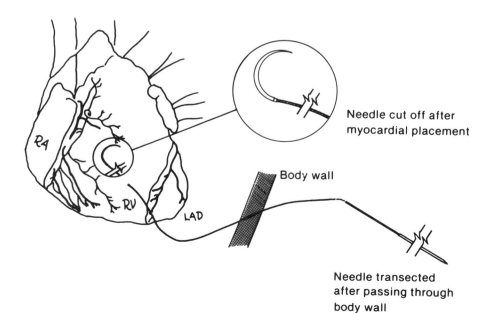

FIG. 3.2. Operative placement of ventricular pacing wire.

A given patient may have no pacing wires at all (straightforward cases only) or may have any of a number of combinations of grounds, atrial wires, and ventricular wires. At the time of operation the surgeon decides which wires might be needed postoperatively. It should be noted that a ground wire can be placed at any time, even in the ICU. If need be, an ordinary EKG skin electrode can be used as a ground.

Most hospitals have conventions that allow the house officer to recognize which wire is which. For example, at some centers, a ventricular wire will be brought to the left side of the chest and an atrial wire will be brought to the right. The ground wire can be recognized because it ends at the skin. Also, since the overall length of the wires is the same, the ground is the wire with more length outside the body.

EMERGENCY PLACEMENT OF PACING WIRES

Emergency placement of pacing wires may be required if bradycardia occurs in an ICU patient who does not have epicardial pacing wires already in place. For this reason the house officer must become familiar with the emergency placement of temporary wires. Two general approaches are available: transvenous and transthoracic.

Transvenous Approach

For placement of a transvenous pacing wire, central venous cannulation is carried out as for intravenous access or central venous pressure (CVP) monitoring (1). The flow-directed temporary transvenous pacing catheter has an inflatable balloon near the tip, just like a Swan-Ganz catheter (Fig. 3.3). The pacing catheter is advanced to CVP position in the right atrium. At this point, the balloon is inflated and the catheter is advanced further. Just as for the Swan-Ganz catheter, the bloodstream carries the balloon and catheter tip through the tricuspid valve into the right ventricle. A sharp further advancement until resistance is felt will engage the tip in the right ventricular trabeculae. At times, the bloodstream will carry the tip through the ventricle to the pulmonary artery; in such a case, withdrawal into the ventricle will be necessary before advancement into the trabeculae. As this is a blind procedure, it is not possible to be absolutely certain of position. (Fluoroscopy is rarely immediately available in the ICU setting.) With some experience, the house officer can get the feel of the procedure. When some (low) spontaneous heart rate is present, the flow-directed catheter can be passed with a reasonable chance of success. If no spontaneous heartbeat at all exists to carry the flow-directed balloon, successful placement is unlikely, as the catheter tends to pass straight through the right atrium into the interior vena cava.

Systems have been described for monitoring the intracardiac EKG by attaching the end of the temporary pacing wire to a 12-lead EKG machine; this can allow identification of position in the ventricle on the basis of EKG characteristics (2). Such monitoring can be cumbersome in emergencies, especially for a beginner. It may be more efficient just to pass the catheter as well as possible and then to connect it to the pacemaker to see if effective pacing is achieved; if not, the catheter is repositioned.

FIG. 3.3. Temporary transvenous pacing catheter.

One common misconception is that a pacing spike on the monitor means that the tip of the catheter is in the heart. This is not true in the slightest. A pacing spike can be seen with the catheter tip *anywhere* in contact with body fluids. It is observation of a wide-complex QRS depolarization following the pacing spike that confirms proper contact with the ventricular myocardium.

Transthoracic Approach

In desperate circumstances, as when no effective heartbeat exists to carry a flow-directed catheter, a transthoracic pacing wire may need to be placed (Fig. 3.4). The right ventricle is punctured by needle via a subxyphoid approach similar to that for pericardiocentesis. A specially designed wire is passed through the needle into the ventricle. Pacing is then instituted as for other catheters. This approach obviously is dangerous and should be used only when no alternative exists.

A

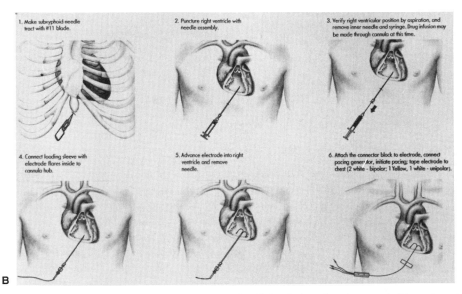

B

FIG. 3.4. A: Temporary transthoracic pacing wire. **B**: Technique for placement. (Reproduced with the permission of Mansfield Scientific, Inc.)

FIG. 3.5. The Paceport Swan-Ganz catheter. Schematic representation shows the pacing wire protruding through the proximal (RV) port and making contact with the right ventricular endocardial surface. (Reproduced with the permission of Baxter Healthcare Corporation.)

The Paceport Swan-Ganz Catheter®

A relatively recent and very useful piece of equipment is the Paceport Swan-Ganz catheter (Baxter Healthcare Corporation; Irvine, CA). This device is a Swan-Ganz catheter that can provide cardiac pacing as well. The concept takes advantage of the fact that, with the Swan-Ganz catheter properly positioned in the pulmonary artery, for most patients a port 19 cm back from the tip of the catheter lies in the right ventricle. A pacing wire specifically designed for passage through this port is used to pace the heart. (See Fig. 3.5.) This device can provide extremely quick access to the right ventricle for pacing. Until pacing is required, the Paceport Swan-Ganz is used just as any other Swan-Ganz catheter for hemodynamic monitoring and cardiac output determination. Use of this model of Swan-Ganz catheter is recommended for circumstances in which the need for pacing appears likely or possible.

THE EXTERNAL TRANSCUTANEOUS (ZOLL) PACEMAKER

It has been known for many years that it is feasible to pace the heart by applying a current between contacts placed on the skin external to the body—by selecting elec-

FIG. 3.6. The external transcutaneous (Zoll) pacemaker. **A:** Electrodes in place in anteroposterior position. **B:** The external console. (Reproduced by permission of ZMI Corporation, 500 W. Cummings Park, Woburn, Massachusetts.)

trode locations that provide a current trajectory that intersects with the heart. In fact, many of the earliest attempts at cardiac pacing involved such systems. These systems fell out of favor—because of their unreliability and, especially, pain associated with pacing—with the advent of fluoroscopy and transvenous pacing systems.

Recent technical advances have made possible reliable and comfortable transcutaneous pacing (3) and have led to a resurgence of this modality. The current system (Zoll) involves two large electrodes placed anteroposteriorly over the left chest. (See

Fig. 3.6.) An external console develops the current applied to the electrodes. The desired heart rate is set on the console, as well as the current output. (Current output of 40–100 mA is usually required, compared to the 1–2 mA required for pacing through a transvenous catheter.) Current level is set so as to provide reliable pacing but minimize pain. The device can be set in a "demand" mode, so that it fires only when bradycardia is occurring.

The house officer should be aware that the mere delivery of the stimulus by the external pacemaker can give the appearance of eliciting a QRS complex while not actually capturing the heart. This is true even of transvenous pacemakers but poses more of a problem by virtue of the high-current, long-duration stimulus required for external pacing. It is crucial to confirm the capture of the heart muscle by feeling a pulse synchronous with the pacemaker spikes or confirming a pressure pulse on the arterial line tracing.

The external transcutaneous pacemaker (Zoll) can provide very quick access to electrical pacing of the heart in emergencies. Transcutaneous pacemakers are now found in most emergency rooms, coronary care units, recovery rooms, and post–cardiac surgery units. The transcutaneous system should be used, when available, in preference to transvenous placement and transthoracic puncture. A brief period of discomfort from pacing is a small price to pay for restoration of a life-supporting heart rate, especially in emergencies where the patient has a reduced level of consciousness. Once stability is restored, a transvenous temporary pacemaker can be placed in a precise manner under fluoroscopic control to provide more reliable and more comfortable pacing.

OPERATING THE PACEMAKER

A commonly used external temporary pacemaker generator is shown in Fig. 3.7. The two knurled knobs on the pacemaker are for securing the ends of the pacing wires. The sense and pace lights indicate what the unit is doing for each beat—sensing or pacing.

Operating Parameters

There are three parameters (set by dials) for the physician to adjust:

1. The **rate** control is self-explanatory. Most units will allow 30–180/min. A reasonable initial setting for a bradycardic patient might be 70 or 80/min. In a patient who is not currently bradycardic but who had shown heart block in the early postoperative period or who is at risk for heart block after myocardial infarction, the rate might be set at 45 or 50/min. In this way, the patient's heart would be allowed to beat spontaneously but would be protected from a life-threatening low rate if heart block should recur.

2. The **output** control allows the current of the pacing stimulus to be adjusted, usually in a range of from 0 to 20 mA. In an emergency, the output should be set to

CONNECTOR TERMINALS

SENSE INDICATOR

BATTERY TEST BUTTON

PACE INDICATOR

ON-OFF SWITCH

BATTERY CARTRIDGE

FIG. 3.7. Ventricular pacemaker (external). (Reproduced with the permission of Medtronic, Inc.)

maximum. Output can, in fact, usually be left at maximum. If the skin is being used as ground, the patient may feel an electric shock at the skin site; this may require turning down the output somewhat. One must, of course, be certain to ascertain that the ventricle is still captured at the lower output setting.

3. The **sensitivity** control allows the sensitivity of the pacemaker to be adjusted. At the lowest sensitivity, labeled "asynchronous," the pacemaker does not listen for a spontaneous heartbeat at all; the pacemaker will fire regularly at the set rate regardless of intrinsic cardiac activity. At full sensitivity, or "demand" setting, the pacemaker will not fire if a spontaneous beat occurs before the scheduled time for the next paced beat. The gradations between these two extremes control the height (in millivolts) that a spontaneous QRS complex must achieve to be recognized by the unit. Usually, the full demand setting will be used. Unfortunately, on most units, the word *demand* does not appear on the dial at the full clockwise position, and this may confuse the house officer. This omission has been rectified on the newer models.

Polarity

The negative pole of the pacemaker should go to the heart and the positive pole should be the ground. This is contrary to what one would expect for an electrical ground. The best way for the house officer to remember this arrangement is to recall that electrons exit from the negative pole of a battery. Better capture occurs when this electron flow hits the heart directly.

Multiple Ventricular Wires

If more than one ventricular wire is present, either can be used as positive or negative. A patient who has discomfort at the skin site with paced beats can be converted to two ventricular leads (if two are available); this will eliminate any discomfort.

Atrial Wires

If the patient has intact atrioventricular (AV) conduction and has atrial wires in place, it is usually preferable to pace atrially. This preserves AV synchrony and atrial kick. If heart block exists, of course, ventricular pacing must be used, as the atrial impulse will not be conducted. Connections for the atrial wires are made similarly to those for the ventricular. Negative goes to the atrium; positive goes to skin ground. If two atrial wires are present, either can be used as positive or negative.

Asynchronous Pacing

If it is ever necessary to use the asynchronous mode, the danger of precipitating ventricular tachycardia is remote. The house officer usually has heard of the R-on-T phenomenon precipitating ventricular tachycardia or ventricular fibrillation. This is a rare phenomenon. If need be, the house officer can pace a patient asynchronously if the demand mode should not work reliably.

The epicardial wires usually function very well in the early postoperative period. Over 7–10 days, however, exit block may occur. Scar tissue and edema at the sites of the wires on the myocardium may insulate the wire electrically from intact muscle. It may become difficult or impossible to capture the myocardium. The R wave heard by the sensing system may diminish in amplitude, leading to improper sensing, with the possibility of the R-on-T phenomenon. In such cases, different combinations of wires may be tried, following the preceding guidelines. One wire may function perfectly when another has exit block or poor R wave.

In case of dysfunction in the pacing system, the house officer must check all components carefully. The wires must be identified correctly and must be connected appropriately, the connections must be tight, and all dials must be set properly. A careful examination and some common sense will usually produce proper pacing.

Sequential Pacing

AV sequential pacing has no role except in complete heart block. If the patient's own conducting system is intact, simple atrial pacing will produce coordinated contraction of both atrial and ventricular chambers, capitalizing on the "atrial kick" to improve cardiac output.

If AV block does exist, the surgeon may choose to use AV sequential pacing. A special external pacemaker is required (Fig. 3.8). This pacemaker paces the atrium

FIG. 3.8. AV sequential pacemaker (external). (Reproduced with the permission of Medtronic, Inc.)

first and then the ventricle after an internal AV delay. An atrial and a ground wire are connected to the atrial output of the unit. A ventricular wire and a ground are connected to the ventricular output of the unit. Two atrial and/or two ventricular wires may be used if present and preferred. The adjustable dials for AV sequential pacing are as follows:

Ventricular rate. This is self-explanatory.
Atrial output. This controls the current delivered to the atrium (0–20 mA).
Ventricular output. This controls the current delivered to the ventricle (0–20 mA).
AV interval. This controls the delay between the atrial and ventricular pacing stimuli. This is usually set in the physiologic range of 150–200 msec.
Ventricular sensitivity. This controls the sensitivity of the ventricular portion of the unit. Again, the full clockwise position represents "demand" mode. (Note that the unit does not sense the atrium at all; accordingly, there is no atrial sensitivity dial.)

The AV sequential unit paces the atrium and ventricle in synchrony. In cases of complete heart block, this can augment cardiac output by capitalizing on the "atrial kick." In an emergency, the house officer's immediate response should be to institute single-chamber ventricular pacing. This should suffice to support life. A transition to dual chamber pacing can be made after stabilization, if required, to augment cardiac output.

The sequential unit does not sense the atrium. In patients who have competing atrial rates, a common phenomenon, the sequential pacemaker can cause atrial fibrilla-

Fig. 3.9. DDD Pacemaker. (Reproduced with permission of Medtronic, Inc.)

tion—essentially by an *atrial* R-on-T phenomenon. This is a serious limitation of the sequential pacemaker.

DDD Pacing

Fully physiologic pacing, which senses and paces both the atrium and the ventricle, has been available in permanent implantable pacemakers for years. This type of pacing is called "DDD" in the international nomenclature.

Despite this sophistication in implantable units, technology has lagged in temporary external units. The sequential pacemakers described earlier do not pace or sense the atrium. Recently, the technology of full, physiologic DDD pacing has become available in external temporary units (4)(Fig. 3.9). Unlike sequential external pacemakers, these units can sense as well as pace the atrium. This can be a tremendous advantage if the atrial rate is irregular and if the AV conduction varies. A heart rate is set for the DDD pacemaker. If a spontaneous atrial beat occurs within the time of the heart rate allotment, the pacemaker does not deliver an atrial stimulus. The unit then listens for a ventricular QRS. If one is sensed, no ventricular pacing stimulus is delivered; if none is sensed, a ventricular pacing stimulus is delivered with the specific AV delay. If no atrial beat occurs within the time of the heart rate allotment, an atrial pacing stimulus is delivered; the unit then listens again for a ventricular QRS. In essence, the unit listens to and/or paces both chambers as required.

The additional settings required for the DDD external unit (above those discussed earlier for the sequential pacemaker) are atrial sensitivity and atrial output. Also, the mode is specified by the house officer; that is, either ventricular (called VVI in the nomenclature), atrial (called AAI), or dual chamber (DDD).

The DDD pacemaker essentially can do everything the simpler pacemakers do and more. These units are making their way into intensive care units and are likely to replace the simpler models. Especially in patients who have heart rates that compete with the paced rate, the DDD pacemakers are optimal, providing AV synchrony despite the beat-to-beat variability of the intrinsic heart rhythm. Atrial R-on-T is prevented.

OVERDRIVE PACING

In addition to their usefulness in bradycardias, external pacemakers can be useful in selected tachyarrhythmias, for so-called overdrive pacing (5,6). The principle involved is to overtake a tachyarrhythmia by pacing the affected chamber faster than the intrinsic tachycardia; upon discontinuation of pacing, the tachyarrhythmia is often found to have been interrupted, with normal sinus rhythm supervening (Fig. 3.10). It may be necessary to overdrive at very rapid rates (e.g., 300/min or more for atrial flutter); special external pacing boxes are available for this purpose.

Overdrive pacing is most effective for supraventricular tachycardias, especially atrial flutter. At some centers, this is the preferred treatment of postoperative atrial

FIG. 3.10. EKG strip demonstrating successful overdrive pacing to terminate supraventricular tachycardia. Note atrial flutter at beginning of strip. The downward spikes in the midportion of the strip represent rapid atrial overdrive pacing. Normal sinus rhythm supervenes when rapid pacing is terminated. (Reproduced with permission from Ref. 7.)

flutter. Even ventricular tachycardia can be treated at times in this way. Only **organized** rhythms can respond; atrial or ventricular fibrillation is never ameliorated by overdrive pacing.

The overdrive pacing technique has serious inherent dangers and should not be undertaken independently by the junior officer; experienced supervision is required.

REFERENCES

1. Vander Salm TJ. *Atlas of bedside procedures.* Boston: Little, Brown; 1979.
2. Schnitzler R, Caracta A, Damato A. "Floating" catheter for temporary transvenous ventricular pacing. *Am J Cardiol* 1973;31:351–354.
3. Zoll PM, Zoll RH, Falk RH, Clinton JE, Eitel DR, Antiman EM. External noninvasive temporary cardiac pacing: clinical trials. *Circulation* 1985;71:937–944.
4. Ferguson TB, Cox JL. Temporary external DDD pacing after cardiac operations. *Ann Thorac Surg* 1991;51:723–732.
5. Fisher J. Pacing for tachycardias. *Resident Staff Physician* July 1980.
6. Waldo A, MacLean W, Karp R, et al. Entrainment and interruption of atrial flutter with atrial pacing: studies in man following open heart surgery. *Circulation* 1977;56:737–745.
7. Harthorne JW. *Intelligence reports in cardiac pacing and electrophysiology* 1984;2:6.

4 The Defibrillator

As discussed in Chapter 2, cardioversion and defibrillation are important techniques for the management of acute disturbances of cardiac rhythm. **Cardioversion** refers to the delivery of a depolarizing electrical impulse *synchronized* with the patient's EKG; **defibrillation** refers to the delivery of a depolarizing impulse *randomly*, without synchronization with the EKG.

The techniques of cardioversion and defibrillation should be within the armamentarium of the house officer, especially if he or she is to treat coronary care or postoperative cardiac patients. All too frequently, unfortunately, the house officer's first responsible application of cardioversion or defibrillation comes during an emergency for which he or she is not prepared. This chapter aims to clarify important basic concepts regarding these techniques. In addition to assimilating the following material, the house officer should spend time with the particular defibrillator used in his own intensive care unit; a review of the instruction manual and a run-through with the controls are important.

GENERAL PRINCIPLES

Figure 4.1 shows a typical defibrillator apparatus. The top portion is an EKG monitor, like those used at the bedside in all ICUs. This monitor displays the EKG on the oscilloscope screen and displays the pulse rate digitally; an EKG printout is available; upper and lower pulse rate alarms can be set for monitoring. This EKG monitor is attached via a standard patient cable to EKG skin electrodes. The lower portion of the apparatus is the cardioverter/defibrillator proper. The charge is selected by dial, displayed digitally, and delivered via the patient paddles.

Because of their greater effectiveness and reliability (1), direct current (DC) units have supplanted earlier alternating current models. When the unit is charged, the DC

47

A

B

FIG. 4.1.

C

FIG. 4.1. A typical defibrillator apparatus. **A:** The assembled apparatus. **B:** Monitor component: 1, oscilloscope; 2, power switch; 3, EKG size control; 4, "beep" volume; 5, EKG strip recorder; 6, EKG recorder mode; 7, battery level indicator; 8, "battery charging" light; 9, EKG lead select; 10, EKG cable connector; 11, QRS flashing light; 12, heart rate (digital); 13, heart rate alarm limits (low and high). **C:** Defibrillator component: 1, power switch; 2, energy select control (in joules); 3, charge button; 4, energy display (in joules); 5, sync switch and flashing light; 6, internal paddle discharge button; 7, battery level indicator; 8, "battery charging" light; 9, connector for internal paddles. (Reproduced with the permission of Physio-Control Corporation.)

charge is stored in a capacitor. The amount of energy stored can be varied, usually from 0 to 400 watt-seconds, or joules. When the unit is fired, the stored charge is delivered from the capacitor to the paddles. The delivery is completed in several milliseconds (Fig. 4.2) (2). Delivery may be made asynchronously or in synchrony with the patient's EKG, at the discretion of the physician (see later). The delivered electrical impulse depolarizes all or most of the muscle fascicles of the heart, interrupts the arrhythmia, and allows normal rhythms to emerge (3).

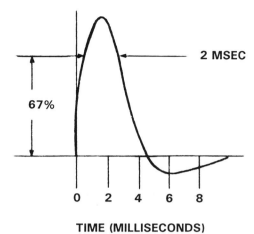

TIME (MILLISECONDS)

FIG. 4.2. Pulse contour of delivered electric shock. (Reproduced with the permission of Mennen Medical, Inc.)

Paddle Position

The cardinal principle regarding paddle position is that the current flowing between the paddles must encompass the heart. Some units incorporate a flat paddle that can be placed underneath the patient's chest; the second paddle goes in front of the heart. This arrangement may use up critical time. More commonly, both paddles are held by hand (Fig. 4.3), one to the right of the sternum just below the clavicle and the second below the left breast and back toward the scapula. This arrangement is convenient and effective.

Electrode paste must be used to obtain good electrical contact between paddles and patient; otherwise, skin burns will result. Gel pads have recently come into favor and serve the same purpose as the older electrode paste. Firm pressure against the patient helps to maximize current delivery. Personnel should step away from the bed to avoid inadvertent shocking. Likewise, electrode jelly should be kept from the paddle handles, as this could form a current path to the operator's hand. A new type of flexible, self-adhesive, disposable paddles (Fast-Patch, R2 pads, and R2 Medical Systems, Niles, Illinois) is available; two such paddles can be left attached to the patient's chest and connected to the defibrillator—for high-risk patients, or those manifesting frequent arrhythmias.

If an elective cardioversion is performed in a conscious patient, analgesia and anesthesia must be effected. Intravenous diazepam (Valium) is effective. An anesthesiologist can be extremely useful to administer Pentothal (or a similar drug), as in the operating room, to obtain complete, brief anesthesia. At the same time, the anesthesiologist can monitor and control respiration and airway. **In critical situations, where vital signs and consciousness are lost, no anesthesia is necessary.** Indeed, no time should be wasted in this setting in giving anesthetic medications.

FIG. 4.3. Standard paddle position. It is best to place the left paddle even more laterally than shown, if possible. (Reproduced with the permission of Physio-Control Corporation.)

Energy Level

The greater the energy delivered, the greater the chance of achieving the desired conversion of rhythm. However, **cardioversion does cause cardiac damage**, and the extent of damage is directly related to the energy level used (3). The electrical energy is dissipated as heat, which injures myocardial cells in the path of the current.

Balancing chance for success against current-mediated cardiac muscle injury requires familiarity with conversion patterns of various rhythms. **Certain rhythms are very sensitive to cardioversion, and low energy levels are likely to bring about conversion; such is the case for atrial flutter and ventricular tachycardia** (4). **Other rhythms are relatively resistant to cardioversion and require higher energy levels; atrial and ventricular fibrillation fall in this category** (4). Further details are given in the discussion of cardioversion of particular arrhythmias.

The other factor that influences choice of energy level is the urgency of the situation. **An elective cardioversion can be done at incremental energies until success is achieved. An emergency defibrillation, on the other hand, can justifiably be performed at a high energy level.**

Most units in current use can provide up to 400 joules for external defibrillation. **For internal defibrillation, much lower energies must be used.** In fact, most units lock out all energy choices beyond 50 joules when connected to internal paddles.

Synchronized Cardioversion or Asynchronous Defibrillation

The house officer should understand when to use synchronized cardioversion and when to use asynchronous defibrillation. The key principle in this decision is that a so-called *vulnerable period*, corresponding to the T wave on EKG, follows ventricular depolarization (Fig. 4.4); delivery of an impulse during the vulnerable period runs the risk of producing ventricular fibrillation.

The cardioverter unit monitors the patient's EKG. When the "synchronized" mode is selected, an electrical circuit in the unit ensures that no impulse is fired during the vulnerable period; instead the impulse is timed to occur during the R wave. When the synchronized mode has been selected and the patient's EKG is being read well by the machine, the "sync" button will flash with each QRS complex detected. Further, the oscilloscope will show a spike on each QRS complex where the machine would have delivered the depolarizing impulse if activated at that time (Fig. 4.5).

Basically, synchronized cardioversion should be used for all rhythms (including atrial fibrillation, atrial flutter, paroxysmal atrial tachycardia, and ventricular tachycardia) **except ventricular fibrillation, for which asynchronous cardioversion must be performed.** The use of synchronized cardioversion will avoid the risk of precipitating ventricular fibrillation while treating a less serious arrhythmia. In ventricular fibrillation, this concern is not relevant. Furthermore, with the constant chaotic electrical and mechanical activity in ventricular fibrillation, no QRS or T waves exist or can be identified.

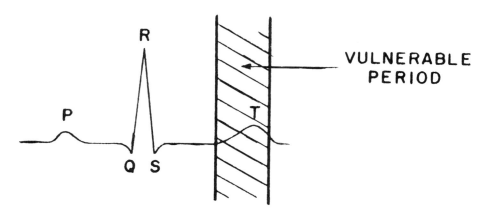

FIG. 4.4 The vulnerable period of the cardiac cycle. (Reproduced with the permission of Mennen Medical, Inc.)

FIG. 4.5. Synchronizer spikes (5) superimposed on the R wave of the EKG.

Now that this basic point regarding synchronous/asynchronous application has been made, some qualifications are in order:

- The risk of inducing ventricular fibrillation with asynchronous cardioversion, although real, is not great. It has been estimated at 2% to 5% (1–3). For this reason, if an arrhythmia for which synchronization would normally be used causes major hemodynamic embarrassment, or if the "sync" apparatus cannot quickly be engaged, asynchronous delivery is justified.
- In ventricular tachycardia it may not be possible for the physician or the machine to identify QRS and T waves, depending on the particular morphology. In this case, asynchronous delivery is acceptable.
- If a patient is discovered in extremis and precise cardiac rhythm cannot be determined rapidly, asynchronous cardioversion is acceptable.

One practical matter deserves emphasis. When synchronized cardioversion is selected, the machine will not deliver the charge at the instant that the paddle controls are pressed; rather, delivery of the charge will be delayed until the appropriate time on the EKG. It is not uncommon to find a junior house officer letting up on the paddle pushbuttons when he or she doesn't see an immediate shock delivered. The house officer concludes the apparatus is not working and may repeat this cycle with continued failure to shock. In fact, the equipment is working appropriately. One must keep the pushbuttons depressed and wait a split second or more for synchronization and shock delivery.

ELECTRICAL CONVERSION OF SPECIFIC RHYTHMS

The overall treatment patterns for specific arrhythmias are covered in Chapter 2. Cardioversion and defibrillation are included in the recommended patterns for many of these rhythms. The particulars of application of cardioversion/defibrillation for specific rhythm disturbances will be covered here.

Cardiac Standstill

Defibrillation is of no use in cardiac standstill. Pacing is required in this circumstance. Occasionally, the question may arise of whether a nearly isoelectric EKG trace represents fine ventricular fibrillation. Defibrillation may be tried if this is considered a real possibility.

Atrial Fibrillation

As discussed in Chapter 2, cardioversion is indicated when acute-onset atrial fibrillation with rapid response causes major compromise of vital signs. Synchronized cardioversion should be performed. Moderate energy levels may at times be required.

Cardioversion is often performed by cardiologists for chronic atrial fibrillation in hopes of improving cardiac output by restoring the atrial kick.

Atrial Flutter

Atrial flutter is often exquisitely sensitive to cardioversion. As little as 10 joules may suffice. Synchronized cardioversion is indicated.

Paroxysmal Atrial Tachycardia

Vagal or pharmacologic maneuvers usually are effective in paroxysmal atrial tachycardia. Synchronized cardioversion may be used if required.

Ventricular Tachycardia

Often ventricular tachycardia does not sustain vital signs. Cardioversion is indicated. Synchronization should be used if possible. If a bizarre configuration does not permit synchronization, asynchronous cardioversion is permissible. Very low energies, even 10 joules at times, often suffice.

Ventricular Fibrillation

The only treatment for ventricular fibrillation is defibrillation. Asynchronous delivery is imperative. High energies are required. Some physicians try 200, then 300, then 400 joules. Others start directly at full energy of 400 joules. We recommend 400 joules as the initial energy. The house officer should remember to turn off the synchronizer circuit if ventricular fibrillation occurs following synchronized cardioversion of another rhythm (5).

COMPLICATIONS

As mentioned briefly earlier, cardioversion does cause myocardial damage. Myocardial enzyme release can be detected in 7% of patients (6). This is the impetus for keeping energy levels as low as possible. In some cases, pulmonary edema or hypotension can be seen as a consequence of cardioversion (4); these phenomena are thought to represent consequences of direct myocardial damage. The recent experience with extensive defibrillation for testing implantable defibrillators is teaching the profession much more about the consequences of the procedures of defibrillation than was previously known (7).

Pulmonary or systemic embolization can be seen when patients with chronic atrial fibrillation are converted electrically. This is the reason for anticoagulating these patients in preparation for cardioversion. Embolization is not a serious risk in cases of acute-onset atrial fibrillation following cardiac or thoracic surgery.

A number of abnormal rhythms may follow cardioversion/defibrillation. The risk of inducing ventricular fibrillation by asynchronous cardioversion has already been discussed. Even with properly synchronized cardioversion, ventricular fibrillation can occur. Ventricular fibrillation is especially likely when the overdigitalized patient is cardioverted (2,4). The house officer should try to avoid cardioversion when digitalis toxicity may be present. Digitalis should be withheld, if possible, prior to cardioversion. If cardioversion must be performed in a patient maintained on digoxin, gradually increasing the energy level until conversion occurs may minimize the risk of precipitating ventricular fibrillation (8,9).

Besides ventricular fibrillation, a number of other arrhythmias may appear following cardioversion/defibrillation. Atrial or ventricular premature beats, changing foci of rhythm, and nodal rhythm are commonly encountered and usually transient. **It is important for the house officer to recognize that asystole may occur following cardioversion.** This is especially common in patients with sick sinus syndrome (10), who, as part of their rhythm disorder, normally manifest both fast and slow supraventricular rhythms. **For this reason, facilities for cardiac pacing should be available when cardioversion is performed.** For the postsurgical cardiac patient, it is best to attach an external pacemaker to the epicardial pacing wires; the pacemaker can then be turned on following cardioversion if required. (See Chapter 3.)

REFERENCES

1. Resnekov L. Present status of electroversion in the management of cardiac dysrhythmias. *Circulation* 1973;47:1356–1363.
2. Mennen-Greatbatch Electronics, Inc. *Operating manual: model 606/F mobile ECG monitor and defibrillator.*
3. National Conference Steering Committee. Standards for cardiopulmonary resuscitation (CPR) and emergency cardiac care. *JAMA* 1974;227:837–868.
4. Lown B, DeSilva RA. The technique of cardioversion. In: Hurst JW, ed. *The heart, arteries, and veins.* New York: McGraw-Hill; 1982:1752–1757.

5. Creed JD, Packard JM, Lambrew CT, Lewis AJ. Defibrillation and synchronized cardioversion. In: McIntyre KM, Lewis AJ, eds. *Textbook of advanced cardiac life support.* Dallas: American Heart Association, 1981:VII-1–VII-7.
6. Elefteriades JA, Handler A, Rosenfield LE, et al. Extensive defibrillation threshold testing for AICD placement does not produce myocardial necrosis. *Eur J Cardiol Pacing Electrophys* 1992;2:A107.
7. Ehsani A, Ewy GA, Sobel BE. Effects of electric countershock on serum creatine phosphokinase (CPK) isoenzyme activity. *Am J Cardiol* 1976;37:12–18.
8. Rubenstein E. *Intensive medical care.* New York: McGraw-Hill; 1971.
9. Mandel WJ. Cardiac arrhythmias. In: Berk JL, Sampliner JE, Artz JS, Vinocur B, eds. *Handbook of critical care.* Boston: Little, Brown; 1976:131–152.
10. Smith WM, Gallagher JJ. Management of arrhythmias and conduction abnormalities. In: Hurst JW, ed. *The heart, arteries and veins.* New York: McGraw-Hill; 1982:557–575.

5 Hemodynamic Monitoring and the Swan-Ganz Catheter

Because ventricular performance in cardiac patients is often abnormal to start with and may be acutely worsened after cardiopulmonary bypass for cardiac surgery, precise hemodynamic monitoring is essential in both the coronary care and postcardiac surgical intensive care units. Monitoring includes assessment of volume status and of cardiac output. Traditional hemodynamic assessment criteria useful in less critically ill patients (such as evaluation of mucous membrane moisture, auscultation of the chest, auscultation of the heart, and examination for peripheral edema) may not suffice for the postinfarct patient or the patient who has undergone open-heart surgery; more precise assessment may be required. Techniques and concepts for this precise hemodynamic assessment form the subject of this chapter.

The following principles apply equally well in the coronary care setting and in the postcardiac surgical intensive care unit.

MONITORING OF VOLUME STATUS

Ideally, for volume status assessment, one would like to know left ventricular end-diastolic pressure (LVEDP). **LVEDP is the ultimate volume status criterion**. It conveys the "state of fullness" of the left ventricle before its contraction begins. In volume depletion, LVEDP will be low. In hypervolemia, LVEDP will be high.

A normal ventricle can pump well without being overfilled. Most normal hearts show an LVEDP of 5–15 mm Hg. Ventricles that require filling pressures of 15–20 mm Hg to pump are beginning to show dysfunction. A ventricle that requires a filling pressure greater than 20 mm Hg in order to pump is severely dysfunctional.

Unfortunately, left ventricular pressure, for practical purposes, cannot be monitored at the bedside. To gain access to the left ventricle requires either cardiac catheterization, with retrograde crossing of the aortic valve under fluoroscopic guidance, or thoracotomy for direct access.

After LVEDP, left atrial mean pressure (LA mean) is the next most accurate index of volume status. It is the mean left atrial pressure that is transmitted to the left ventricle through the open mitral valve in diastole. Unfortunately, the left atrium is likewise relatively inaccessible. In a very sick heart, the surgeon may leave a catheter (an "LA line") indwelling in the left atrium following cardiac surgery. This provides an excellent guide for volume management. Normal LA mean pressures, like normal LVEDP pressures, range between 5 and 15 mm Hg. LA lines, however, pose a number of serious hazards. Air or particulate embolism to the left side of the circulation (especially to the head or the coronary arteries) may occur while the catheter is in place; also, the LA catheter is removed percutaneously, and bleeding can occur from the atrial site.

Thus direct bedside monitoring of the left side of the heart is not commonly used at present. The right side, however, is easily accessible: the great veins (subclavian and jugular) can be cannulated and lead directly to the right heart. Normal diastolic

FIG. 5.1. Discrepancy between right and left heart pressures. Wedge pressure reflects left heart function (see text). Pressures represented here were measured in patients with acute myocardial infarction. (Reproduced with permission from Ref. 16.)

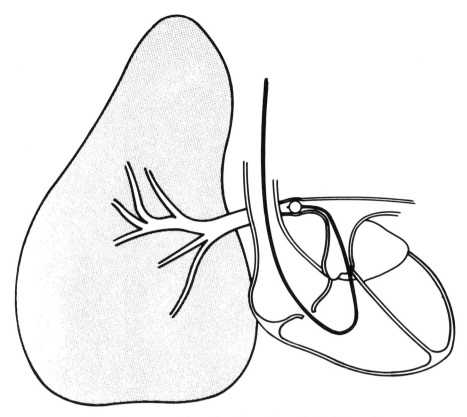

FIG. 5.2. Schematic representation of the Swan-Ganz catheter in the pulmonary artery.

pressures in the right ventricle range from 5 to 10 mm Hg, slightly lower than in the left. Systolic pressures in the right ventricle, of course, are considerably lower than in the left: 25–35 mm Hg, as opposed to systemic pressures of about 120 mm Hg. It is, however, the diastolic pressures that reflect volume state, or "preload." Right atrial mean pressures range normally from 5 to 10 mm Hg. The RA mean pressure is identical to the well-known CVP (central venous pressure).

Thus left heart pressure is what we need to know, but the left heart is inaccessible. The right heart is accessible. It is well known, however, that right heart pressures, especially in the face of serious illness, do not accurately reflect left heart pressures (1–4); compliance, contractility, and afterload may differ significantly between the right and left sides of the circulation. Figure 5.1 demonstrates the scatter between CVP and left heart pressures.

An indwelling pulmonary arterial (Swan-Ganz) catheter solves this dilemma. It allows us to assess **left**-sided pressures by **right** heart catheterization (Fig. 5.2). The Swan-Ganz catheter is introduced through a great vein into the cavity of the right heart, passes through the chambers of the right heart, and is carried by blood flow through the pulmonic valve into the pulmonary artery. The catheter carries an inflatable balloon near its tip. With the catheter tip in the pulmonary artery, the balloon can be inflated. With the balloon inflated, the bloodstream carries the catheter tip distally along the pulmonary artery until the balloon impacts in a branch of the pulmonary artery. This is referred to as *wedging*. Herein lies the key. With the catheter wedged (Fig. 5.3), the tip is no longer exposed to pressure from the right heart: the inflated balloon blocks forward transmission of pressure. The tip is exposed to the blood beyond the balloon in the distal radicles of the pulmonary artery. Through the capillaries of the pulmonary artery, these radicles communicate with the originating radicles of the pulmonary veins, which in turn communicate directly, without valves, with the left atrium. **Thus with the catheter wedged, the pressure seen at the tip, the so-called** *pulmonary capillary wedge pressure (PCWP),* **approximates the LA mean pressure**.

Wedging the catheter carries some risk (see later) and is somewhat temperamental: a given catheter may not wedge at all times desired. When not wedged, the catheter can be used to read pulmonary artery diastolic pressure (PADP). Although pulmonary

FIG. 5.3. Schematic representation of the principle by which Swan-Ganz catheter provides left heart information. When the balloon is inflated (**A**), the tip is isolated from forward pressure from the right ventricle. As in the "closed-pipe" analogy (**B**), reading of the transmitted left atrial pressure is possible. (Reproduced with permission from Ref. 16.)

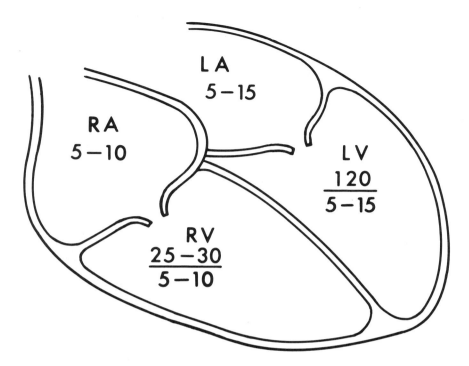

FIG. 5.4. Normal pressures in various cardiac chambers.

arterial pressure is somewhat influenced by right heart function, toward the end of diastole the pressure in the pulmonary artery equilibrates fairly well with the pressure in the pulmonary veins and left atrium. PADP can be used to approximate PCWP when necessary. PADP approximates PCWP much better than does CVP. PADP is most discrepant with PCWP in the presence of lung disease with pulmonary vascular changes. In this case, right-sided pressures, including CVP and PADP, may be severely elevated, whereas PCWP is normal.

To recap: LVEDP is what we need to know. LA mean pressure accurately approximates LVEDP. The Swan-Ganz catheter is helpful because PCWP, which it measures, approximates LA mean. PADP approximates PCWP. CVP and RA mean, which approximate RVEDP, may not accurately reflect left heart filling pressures in the seriously ill patient. This may be summarized as follows:

$$\text{CVP} \sim \text{RA mean} \sim \text{RVEDP} \lesssim \text{PADP} \sim \text{PCWP} \sim \text{LA mean} \sim \text{LVEDP}$$

The correlation between left- and right-sided pressures is lost in cardiac and/or pulmonary disease, and the pulmonary artery catheter becomes essential for measuring left-sided pressures.

Furthermore, it should be pointed out that PADP approximates PCWP but is usually 2–5 mm Hg higher (after all, blood must flow forward into the lung). PCWP approximates LA mean pressure, but it also is usually 2–5 mm Hg higher (after all, blood must flow forward out of the lung).

Thus the pulmonary arterial indwelling catheter provides the best available index of the volume status of the left ventricle short of cardiac catheterization or direct exposure. Figure 5.4 summarizes normal pressures in the various heart chambers.

USE OF THE SWAN-GANZ CATHETER

Particular aspects regarding use of the Swan-Ganz catheter will be addressed next.

Pressure Tracings at Different Catheter Positions

The house officer who places or uses the Swan-Ganz catheter must be familiar with the pressure wave forms in the different chambers of the heart (Fig. 5.5). It is instructive to consider the tracings that one will see as the catheter is advanced through the chambers of the heart during placement.

In the great vein (jugular or subclavian), a typical CVP trace is seen. This is a low-amplitude, uneven sawtooth wave form. The house officer will recall from physiology that this wave form actually includes the a, c, and v waves of the venous pulse. The a wave corresponds to atrial contraction; c, to ventricular contraction with bulging of the atrioventricular valve; and v, to entry of blood into the atrium during late systole (5). As the catheter passes to the right atrium, the same low-amplitude, uneven, sawtooth wave form continues to be seen. (There are no valves between the great veins and the right atrium.)

As the catheter is advanced through the tricuspid valve to the right ventricle, a marked change in the wave form occurs. One now sees a high-amplitude, smooth, regular wave form representing ventricular contraction. Important characteristics are that there is no dicrotic notch and that, at its lowest, the wave nears baseline (0 mm Hg).

As the catheter is advanced through the pulmonary valve into the pulmonary artery, two significant changes in wave form occur: (1) There is now a dicrotic notch, representing pulmonary valve closure, after the peak of systole, and (2) the baseline no longer comes close to zero, because the pulmonary valve serves to maintain diastolic pressure in the pulmonary arterial tree.

As the catheter is advanced further, into the wedge position, one sees again a low-amplitude, irregular, sawtooth wave form representing the wedge tracing. Again, a, c, and v waves can be discerned on close inspection. The mean pressure in this position is the one that best approximates LA mean pressure.

The house officer must become thoroughly familiar with these characteristic tracings. This is important initially in placing the catheter and subsequently in interpreting the tracings. The house officer should become familiar with the pulmonary arterial and wedge pressure tracings of each patient under his care. A change in trace should raise suspicion of dislodgement. It is not uncommon for the nurse to report a very low

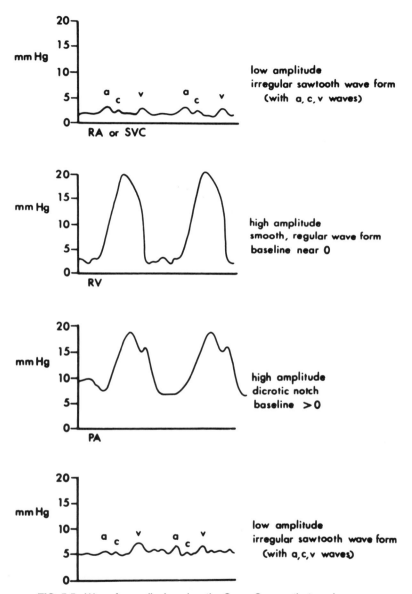

FIG. 5.5. Wave forms displayed as the Swan-Ganz catheter advances.

PADP that in fact represents RVEDP, after a Swan-Ganz catheter has been inadvertently withdrawn to the right ventricle. This mistake can lead to serious overtransfusion.

Physical Characteristics of the Swan-Ganz Catheter

Figure 5.6 illustrates the construction of the Swan-Ganz catheter. Figure 5.6A presents an overall schematic diagram of the catheter. The distal lumen leads to the opening at the tip (in the pulmonary artery). The proximal lumen leads to an opening 30 cm back from the tip (corresponding to the right atrium). The balloon inflation lumen leads to the balloon near the tip of the catheter (this lumen does not connect to the bloodstream). The particular catheter depicted is thermodilution-equipped to allow measurement of cardiac output (see below); for this purpose, an electrical connector leads via a wire to a thermistor 4 cm from the tip of the catheter (6). Figure 5.6B shows a cross-section of a cut catheter. Figure 5.6C shows the distal opening at the tip of the catheter and the inflated balloon.

In general, the distal opening and lumen are used for pressure monitoring (PADP or PCWP). The proximal opening, which lies in the right atrium, can be used for CVP monitoring, for infusion of fluids or drips, or for rapid injection during cardiac output determination. The balloon lumen transmits air to and from the balloon for inflation and deflation.

It should be noted that some Swan-Ganz catheters are made with an additional proximal lumen (making four lumens overall), which may be used for continuous CVP monitoring or fluid or drug administration.

Instrumentation: Transducers, Monitors, and Techniques

The transducer translates the pressure wave form into an electrical signal that is amplified by the monitor and displayed on the oscilloscope screen. A digital read-out system selects and displays systolic, diastolic, or mean pressures from the graphic (analog) signal. The house officer should become familiar with the method of zeroing and calibrating the transducer and monitor system. This technique varies from system to system. In general, the system is "zeroed" (or "balanced") by opening the transducer to air and adjusting the monitor to read atmospheric pressure as zero. The system is calibrated by supplying a known signal and adjusting the gain until exactly the appropriate reading is obtained. This may be done electrically on the basis of a predetermined "calibration factor" for each transducer, or even more accurately by mechanical means—by applying a known pressure from an ordinary blood pressure cuff to the transducer and adjusting gain until the desired reading is obtained. Exact zeroing and balancing practices vary from unit to unit. Some disposable systems are so accurately produced that only zeroing need be done. (Calibration is unnecessary because of very close electrical tolerances in manufacture.) Before taking important readings, the house officer and nurse should confirm zero and calibration together according to local practice.

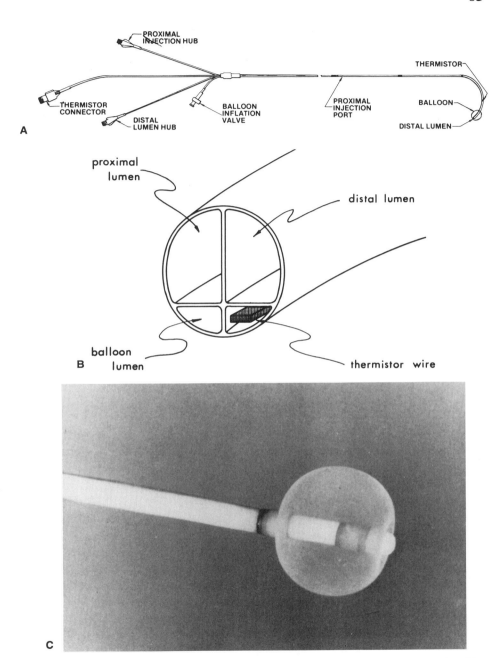

FIG. 5.6. Physical characteristics of the Swan-Ganz catheter. **A:** Schematic representation. (Reproduced with the permission of Edwards Laboratories, Inc.) **B:** Cross-section. **C:** Tip with balloon inflated. (Reproduced with permission from Ref. 16.)

The system must give a crisp, accurate trace. Figure 5.7 indicates sites where leaks, bubbles, or occlusions can impair trace quality and accuracy (7).

The patient must be placed supine for pressure measurements. Without this standardization, pressures will not be able to be interpreted consistently.

The transducer must be located at approximately left atrial level. In some ICUs this is done by placing the transducer on a box on the patient's mattress. In other units the transducer is firmly secured on a pole at the side of the bed. Left atrial level can be approximated at midchest. For every centimeter that the transducer level is off the appropriate height, measured filling pressures will be off accordingly. **Too high a transducer will lead to falsely low pressures; too low a transducer, to falsely high pressures** (1).

It is not at all uncommon for the house officer to make decisions on the basis of filling pressures that are recorded with poorly balanced transducers, with the patient not squarely supine, with the transducer inappropriately positioned, or with the catheter not in the pulmonary artery at all. If a decision regarding intervention is to be made, the house officer should not accept filling pressures as reported by phone or as listed on the day sheet, but must go to the bedside, evaluate the trace, assess patient and transducer position, confirm calibration, and only then read pressures and act on them.

The house officer should recall that electronic systems read pressures in mm Hg. Multiplying by 1.36 will give the equivalent in cm H_2O. Water manometers used for CVP monitoring, of course, read in cm H_2O.

TROUBLE SHOOTING THE PRESSURE MONITORING SYSTEM

FIG. 5.7. Sites of possible malfunction in pressure monitoring system. (Reproduced with permission from Ref. 15.)

Abnormalities of the Swan-Ganz Trace

Three abnormalities in the pulmonary artery trace may confuse the house officer (Fig. 5.8). A damped trace lacks the crisp contours of the properly functioning system. Readings cannot be relied upon in this setting. Eliminating a bubble, flushing the catheter, or correcting a kinked tubing may improve the trace and allow accurate readings.

Occasionally, physical characteristics of the system produce an overcrisp tracing with so-called whip artifact (see Fig. 5.8). In such a case, unfavorable interaction of system components exaggerates pressure fluctuations, impairing parameter measurement. It may be necessary to replace the catheter to remedy this situation.

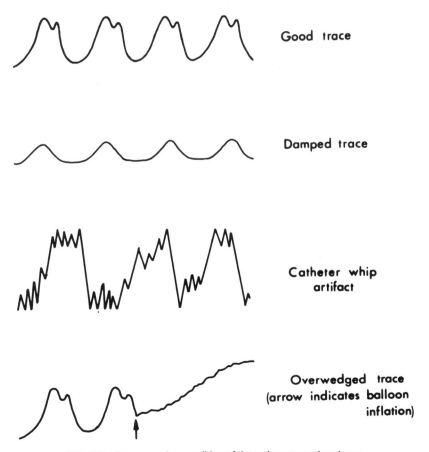

Good trace

Damped trace

Catheter whip artifact

Overwedged trace (arrow indicates balloon inflation)

FIG. 5.8. Common abnormalities of the pulmonary artery trace.

In some cases, with balloon inflation, an "overwedged" trace occurs (Fig. 5.8). In such a case, an initially proper wedge trace rises steadily to very high pressure levels. The exact mechanism is not known (5), but the phenomenon is thought to be related to occlusion of the distal lumen opening by the balloon. Repeating balloon inflation slowly with very small volumes of air may rectify the trace.

Complications of the Swan-Ganz Catheter

The most dreaded complication of Swan-Ganz catheterization is pulmonary artery perforation (8). Fortunately, this frequently lethal complication is uncommon; its occurrence can be minimized by inflating the balloon with no more than 1.5 ml and terminating inflation as soon as the transition to a wedge trace occurs. Inflation should always be done gently. Overinflating can tear the pulmonary artery. Special care must be used in patients with pulmonary artery hypertension, who are more vulnerable to pulmonary rupture. It is important as well never to leave the balloon inflated long-term. Even with the balloon deflated, a continuous wedge trace may appear. This is thought to represent distal migration of the catheter tip as a result of expansion from body heat. Whenever a continuous wedge trace is seen, the catheter should be withdrawn until a pulmonary artery trace reappears. Some centers limit wedging to just once or several times daily because of the danger of perforation. With occasional wedging, the correlation between PADP and PCWP can be determined and PCWP predicted accurately from PADP in the interim.

Arrhythmias are seen commonly during placement of the Swan-Ganz catheter. PVCs are seen almost universally when the tip traverses the right ventricle. Ectopy usually quiets down when the pulmonary arterial position is reached. As discussed in Chapter 2, a catheter that lies just beyond the pulmonary valve and flips in and out of the right ventricle may cause paroxysms of severe ventricular ectopy. Occasionally, even with the tip of the catheter located well distally in the pulmonary artery, the loop in the ventricle may cause ectopy; it may on occasion be necessary to remove the catheter in such an instance.

Pulmonary infarction at the site of the catheter tip may be seen radiographically with some frequency (Fig. 5.9). As the catheter is only 2 mm in diameter, the occluded or thrombosed pulmonary arterial radicle is usually small; any infarction is usually not of clinical significance. If the balloon were inadvertently left inflated, its 13-mm diameter could occlude a major pulmonary arterial branch and cause significant parenchymal injury.

Very frequently the catheter quickly becomes coated with a thin layer of fibrin. Clot commonly forms in the great vein through which the catheter passes, but significant related clinical problems are rare.

On occasion, the balloon at the tip of the catheter may rupture from overdistension or overuse. This may manifest as loss of resistance to syringe inflation or as blood return into the balloon lumen. In this instance, care must be taken to avoid continued instillation of air into the pulmonary artery.

FIG. 5.9. Radiographic appearance of pulmonary infarction distal to a Swan-Ganz catheter. (Reproduced with permission from Ref. 16.)

Influence of Respiration

Filling pressures can be read most accurately in a patient who is not breathing spontaneously—that is, in a patient on a ventilator who is sedated or paralyzed. This is the state of affairs in the critical first few hours after cardiac surgery. In fact, it has been suggested that temporary paralysis and mechanical ventilation be induced whenever filling pressures must be known unequivocally and with complete accuracy (9).

With mechanical ventilation, the measured filling pressures, either PADP or PCWP, vary with the respiratory cycle (Fig. 5.10). Pressures will increase during inspiration, as some of the positive endobronchial pressure is distributed intrathoracically. The correct pressures are those between inspirations.

Likewise, high values of positive end-expiratory pressure (PEEP) can affect pressure readings. Approximately one-third of endobronchial pressure is distributed intrathoracically (10,11). The house officer can confirm this at the bedside in several of his patients. Thus, as an approximation, one can subtract one-third of the PEEP value from the observed pressures. That is, a patient on 15 cm H_2O PEEP whose monitor records a PADP of 15 mm Hg has real PADP of approximately 15 mm Hg minus one-third of 15 cm H_2O, or 10 mm Hg. A more precise true filling pressure can be read by taking the patient off the ventilator for a few seconds (1,10,11). This maneuver can be reserved for patients on high amounts of PEEP. The 5 cm H_2O PEEP used routinely has very little effect on observed filling pressures.

If the patient is breathing spontaneously, the filling pressure trace will again vary cyclically with respiration (see Fig. 5.10). In this case, intrathoracic pressure and observed filling pressure will fall with inspiration. This effect can bring observed filling pressures abnormally low. For this reason, we usually read filling pressures just before inspiration in spontaneously breathing patients.

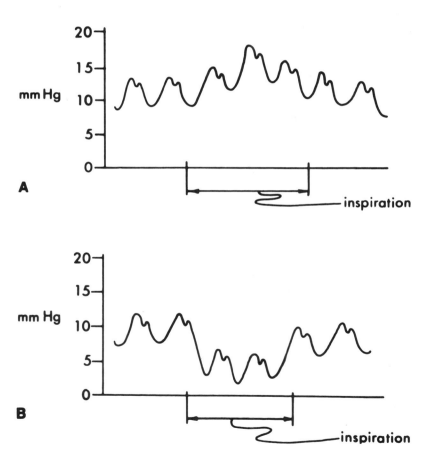

FIG. 5.10. Influence of respiration on the Swan-Ganz trace. (**A**) Positive pressure ventilation. (**B**) Spontaneous (negative pressure) ventilation.

Thus **for either the positive pressure-ventilated or the spontaneously respiring patient, filling pressures are best read just before inspiration** (1,9). In the positive pressure-ventilated patient, inspiration will falsely raise pressures, and in the spontaneously respiring patient, inspiration will falsely lower pressures. With practice, the house officer can learn to correlate the continuously updated digital readout on the monitor with the phasic variation of the graphic pressure display.

Influence of State of Sedation

With very rare exceptions, the filling pressures may vary from hour to hour but do not change significantly from minute to minute. An acute rise in PADP or PCWP is often mistaken by the house officer for a significant alteration in myocardial performance when really it represents the patient's beginning to awaken. As a patient emerges from sedation, vasomotor tone increases and observed PADP may increase dramatically in seconds or minutes. This does not represent myocardial dysfunction. Once it is confirmed that the patient's CNS function is intact, the best treatment may be to sedate the patient again. Diuretics or vasodilators are **not** indicated for changes in pressures seen upon awakening.

Obtaining, transducing, recording, and interpreting pulmonary artery pressures thus involve a complex process with many potential sites of error. Only through thorough understanding and practical experience can house officers ensure that they are obtaining accurate information on which to base therapeutic decisions.

Use of the Swan-Ganz Catheter for Specific Hemodynamic Problems

The Swan-Ganz catheter can diagnose and differentiate between acute mitral regurgitation and acute ventricular septal defect. Patients in the coronary care unit following myocardial infarction who demonstrate low cardiac output or cardiogenic shock may have isolated left ventricular myocardial insufficiency. On the other hand, these patients may have sufficient myocardial reserve but suffer from one of two serious acute mechanical defects: mitral regurgitation or ventricular septal rupture (12). In acute mitral regurgitation from ischemic rupture or dysfunction of the mitral papillary apparatus, regurgitation from the left ventricle into the left atrium impairs left ventricular output and causes pulmonary vascular congestion. In ventricular septal rupture from ischemic transmural septal necrosis, regurgitation from the left to the right ventricle impairs left ventricular output and overwhelms the right heart. Each of these conditions causes a systolic murmur. Each condition is very poorly tolerated, and each requires urgent diagnosis and surgical treatment.

The Swan-Ganz catheter allows diagnosis of and discrimination between these two acutely life-threatening complications of myocardial infarction. **In acute mitral regurgitation, the wedge trace shows a "v wave" representing the regurgitant flow into the left atrium** (Fig. 5.11). The height of the v wave can be read from the monitor and to some extent reflects the severity of the regurgitation.

FIG. 5.11. Pulmonary artery (PA) trace in a patient with mitral insufficiency. The v wave can be distinguished from an ordinary PA systolic wave by the fact that it occurs later with regard to the QRS complex. (Reproduced with permission from Ref. 16.)

In acute ventricular septal rupture, an oxygen step-up is seen between the right atrium and the pulmonary artery. Blood sampled from the distal port (in the pulmonary artery) shows an oxygen saturation significantly higher than that of blood sampled from the proximal part (in the right atrium). This is diagnostic of an abnormal communication between the right and left heart chambers.

The Swan-Ganz catheter is also useful in the diagnosis of hemodynamically significant pulmonary embolus (3). (See also Chapter 18.) Minor embolus insufficient to cause circulatory changes will not be detected. With major embolus, mechanical obstruction of the pulmonary arterial system and especially vasoactive amine-mediated constriction of the pulmonary arteries result in an acute elevation in pulmonary vascular resistance. As a consequence, all right heart pressures, including CVP and pulmonary artery systolic and diastolic pressures, rise, reflecting the strain on the right heart; PCWP, reflecting left heart function, remains unchanged. It is fair to state that **acute pulmonary embolus is not the cause of new-onset hypotension unless a rise is seen in CVP and pulmonary artery systolic and diastolic pressures**.

The Swan-Ganz catheter is useful as well in the diagnosis of cardiac tamponade (3). **In tamponade, one sees equilibration of all pressures—RA mean, RVEDP, PADP, and PCWP—to a high value, usually near 20 mm Hg** (Fig. 5.12).

FIG. 5.12. Characteristic pressures in cardiac tamponade. Note the equalization of RA mean, RVEDP, PADP, and PCWP near 20 mm Hg.

Limitations of the Swan-Ganz Catheter

Finally, recent evidence points out that even the PCWP may not accurately reflect LA mean in the postoperative cardiac patient or other critically ill patients (10). Chronic obstructive pulmonary disease, with pulmonary hypertension, can render even the PCWP discrepant from LA mean. Likewise, pulmonary venous spasm, postulated to occur in acute respiratory distress syndrome (ARDS), may interrupt the continuity of the vascular channel between pulmonary artery and left atrium; estimation of left-sided pressures by pulmonary artery wedging is predicated on this continuity. It is likely that use of direct LA lines for postoperative patients with critically sick hearts will continue.

Evidence has shown as well (13) that another limitation of the Swan-Ganz catheter is that filling pressures do not correlate well with left-ventricular end-diastolic volume (LVEDV), especially in critically ill and postoperative patients. LVEDV is probably the ultimate measure of preload state. ECHO measurements are being used increasingly to provide direct information regarding LVEDV. (See also Chapter 11.)

MONITORING OF CARDIAC OUTPUT

The experienced clinician combines multiple pieces of information into a gestalt that reflects adequacy of cardiac output (CO). We will discuss now the factors that enter into this assessment.

Clinical Criteria

The operating surgeon can tell much about myocardial performance from the look and feel of the heart after coming off cardiopulmonary bypass. The surgeon can tell a sluggishly contractile heart from one beating strongly and effortlessly. He or she can tell by watching the ventricles and feeling the pulmonary artery whether the heart is functioning at normal filling pressures or whether it is beginning to fail and to distend. Thus by the time the chest is closed, the surgeon and the surgical team have a good idea of the state of cardiac function. This information should be conveyed to the house officer who will be caring for the patient. Along with this information should be conveyed the measured details at the completion of the procedure before transfer from the operating room. The BP, CO, PADP, PCWP, and LA mean (if measured) at completion should be relayed. The type and rate of continuous infusions should be conveyed as well. This information will give the house officer a baseline for evaluation of hemodynamics in the ICU.

We will consider now the means available to the house officer in the ICU cardiac output assessment.

Blood pressure is, of course, an important parameter. If BP is low (say, less than 90 mm Hg systolic), it is likely, though not entirely certain, that CO is low. If BP is well maintained, it is likely that CO is satisfactory, though again, not always so. **BP**

does not directly reflect CO because resistance of the systemic circuit (systemic vascular resistance, SVR) may vary. As will be recalled from physiology, the counterpart of Ohm's law is the familiar relation $BP = CO \times SVR$. BP may be maintained by adequacy of CO or by high SVR. In fact, it is possible after cardiac surgery to have a very high BP from a marked elevation in resistance with very little effective CO.

Urine output is another excellent parameter. By and large, a urine output of 30 ml/h or more implies adequate renal perfusion and, by consequence, adequate CO. Several conditions in the postoperative cardiac patient may, however, invalidate this criterion. Most heart-lung machine perfusion regimens include mannitol or furosemide (Lasix) and may artificially produce a high urine flow even in the face of a low CO. The same holds true for osmotic diuresis from hyperglycemia, which is seen commonly after cardiac operations. These effects may linger for hours after return of the patient to the ICU. **In the absence of the effects of diuretic agents, urine output is a good indicator of adequacy of CO.**

Extremity perfusion is another important criterion. By and large, **warm extremities indicate an adequate CO.** It does, however, take time for the extremities to warm after the systemic hypothermia and vasoconstriction of cardiopulmonary bypass. Also, vascular disease of the lower extremities, so common in cardiac surgical patients, can preclude warming of the feet and legs even if CO is good.

Level of consciousness is another useful criterion. **A patient who is awake and alert is perfusing the brain adequately and is therefore likely to have satisfactory CO.** Obtundation and restlessness are usually seen in low-output states. However, following cardiac surgery, several hours are usually required for full emergence from anesthesia; thus this criterion is not usually useful in the immediate postoperative period.

The experienced clinician can assess the strength of cardiac contraction by feeling a peripheral pulse. In the postoperative cardiac patient, who will have an indwelling arterial line, the strength of the peripheral pulse corresponds to the area under the arterial pressure curve (Fig. 5.13). The area under this curve indicates, roughly, the effectiveness of stroke volume, and thus CO. In fact, numerous formulas have been devised to allow precise estimation of CO from the arterial pressure curve (14). A narrow pulse curve or one with a low peak subtends a small area and indicates a low stroke volume; a brisk, wide pressure trace reflects an effective stroke volume.

Objective Criteria

The experienced clinician, by taking all such factors into account, gets a reasonable idea of the CO of the patient. It has been demonstrated that such clinical criteria do correlate with objectively measured CO (15). With some experience, the house officer as well will begin to formulate his or her own impression of CO. Even the most experienced clinician, however, needs to confirm this impression by objective measurements. **The Swan-Ganz catheter allows quantitative measurement of CO via two means: mixed venous oxygen determination and thermodilution.**

normal

low peak   narrow pulse

FIG. 5.13. Characteristic arterial pressure curves.

By providing access to the pulmonary artery, **the Swan-Ganz catheter permits sampling of mixed venous blood for measurement of mixed venous pO_2 (pvO_2).** Blood returning to the right atrium comes in streams that have varying O_2 content. Blood currents from the superior and inferior venae cavae and the coronary sinus usually have had different amounts of oxygen extracted. Coronary sinus blood is always quite desaturated. For this reason, to sample venous blood from the right atrium does not accurately reflect overall oxygen extraction by the body as a whole. These different currents of venous blood mix in the right atrium are further mixed in the right ventricle and are then ejected into the pulmonary artery. Blood in this artery is generally quite uniform in its O_2 saturation and is generally considered to represent true "mixed venous blood." This blood can be sampled by aspirating from the **distal** port of the Swan-Ganz catheter.

When arterial blood is adequately oxygenated, pvO_2 allows indirect assessment of CO. If CO is poor, tissues extract more oxygen from each cycle of passing blood, and pvO_2 is low. If CO is good, the tissues extract less oxygen per cycle, and pvO_2 is high. (This is the basis of CO estimation by the Fick principle.) Thus pvO_2 is directly related to CO. Table 5.1 is a rough guide for the assessment of cardiac output from pvO_2 (10,16,17). We rarely see a pvO_2 of 40 in postoperative cardiac surgical patients. We are pleased by a pvO_2 in the high 30s, whereas pvO_2s in the 20s imply that something is seriously amiss and must be rectified.

A new generation of Swan-Ganz catheters (18) incorporates a fiberoptic oximetry system in the catheter itself, allowing continuous bedside monitoring of mixed venous oxygen saturation. The information that was previously available by periodic

Table 5.1. *Assessment of CO from pvO$_2$*

pvO$_2$ (mm Hg)	CO
35 to 40	Excellent
30 to 35	Good
25 to 30	Fair
20 to 25	Poor
20 or below	Non-life-supporting

sampling of mixed venous blood is now available continuously, "on line," in "real time," without withdrawal of blood. The normal range for saturation of the mixed venous blood is 60% to 80% (corresponding to vpO$_2$ of 30–50 mm Hg). Many hospitals have not yet bought into this technology, as it is not clear that continuous mixed venous saturation monitoring is clinically superior to conventional periodic sampling of mixed venous blood for blood gas analysis.

The Swan-Ganz catheter also allows calculation of cardiac output by thermodilution (Fig. 5.14). Not all Swan-Ganz catheters are designed for measurement of CO; those designed for this purpose are appropriately labeled. CO measurement is done by thermodilution; the Stewart-Hamilton principle is applied, with a cold so-

FIG. 5.14. Thermodilution cardiac output computer. (These computers are being phased out as free-standing units, being incorporated into the main monitors used at the bedside in intensive care units.)

lution being the indicator measured (19). Cold saline is injected into one of the proximal ports (emptying into the right atrium). A thermistor near the tip of the catheter (in the pulmonary artery) monitors the blood temperature curve as the cold bolus is ejected by the right heart. It is assumed that right and left heart CO values are the same—that is, that there are no right-to-left intracardiac communications. The faster the decay of the cold bolus seen at the thermistor, the better the CO. A computer connected electrically to the thermistor does the calculus involved and digitally displays a CO in liters per minute.

Modern thermodilution systems actually display the thermodilution curve, the graph of temperature over time (Fig. 5.15). This can be helpful in evaluating the accuracy of a given measurement. "Bad curves" may have a double hump, or no hump, or an exaggerated undulation. The cardiac output is inversely proportional to the area under the curve. Tricuspid insufficiency characteristically gives a low, flat curve and underestimates the cardiac output due to reverse flow of some of the "cold" indicator backward into the right atrium (20). Tricuspid insufficiency is quite common in critically ill patients, who often have volume overload with resultant dilatation of the tricuspid annulus.

The house officer should be aware that these thermodilution CO readings, though displayed digitally to two decimal places, are of limited accuracy. They

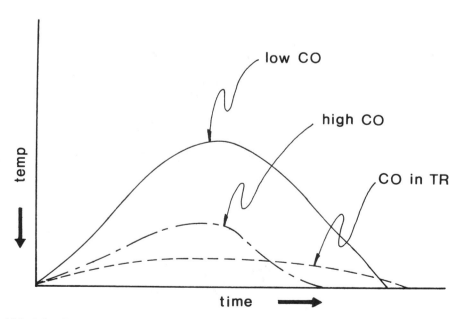

FIG. 5.15. Thermodilution cardiac output (CO) curves (temperature vs time, as "read" by the thermistor at the tip of the catheter). Cardiac output is inversely proportional to the area under the curve (Stewart-Hamilton equation). Curves shown are Normal CO, High CO, Low CO, Low, flat curve of tricuspid insufficiency (which underestimates actual CO).

are very susceptible to error through changes in speed of injection of the bolus, insufficient cooling of the injectate, and many other factors (4,21,22). It is quite common to see a wide scatter among different runs. Three runs should be averaged whenever a CO reading is required.

At times, pvO_2 proves more consistently reliable than thermodilution CO. Furthermore, pvO_2 reflects not only the mechanical pumping effectiveness of the heart, but also the adequacy of CO in meeting the metabolic requirements of the body. Many surgical patients have greatly increased CO needs. If CO meets metabolic requirements, pvO_2 will be normal; if CO falls behind metabolic requirements, pvO_2 will fall, as more oxygen is extracted peripherally by the tissues.

Thermodilution provides an assessment of CO in liters per minute. For purposes of comparison, **the cardiac index is obtained by dividing CO by body surface area** (average areas range from 1.4 to 2.0 m²), giving a value in liters per minute per square meter. **For a postoperative cardiac patient, an index of 3.0 represents excellent CO.** Mild reduction in CO is associated with an index in the range of 2.2–3.0. **Moderately severe reduction is reflected by an index between 1.5 and 2.2. Extremely severe depression of CO is present when the index falls below 1.5** (19). For postoperative cardiac patients, outputs in this range correlate with a high probability of cardiac death (15).

The house officer should keep in mind that the objective criteria of CO are not totally accurate. By integrating the clinical criteria described earlier with the objective measures of CO, the clinician can gain a well-substantiated assessment of cardiac performance.

REFERENCES

1. O'Quin R, Marmi J. Pulmonary artery occlusion pressure: clinical physiology, measurement, and interpretation. *Am Rev Respir Dis* 1983;128:319–326.
2. Samii K, Conseiller C, Viars P. Central venous pressure and pulmonary wedge pressure: a comparative study in anesthetized surgical patients. *Arch Surg* 1976;111:1122–1125.
3. Buchbinder N, Ganz W. Hemodynamic monitoring: invasive techniques. *Anesthesiology* 1976; 45:146–155.
4. Civetta J. Pulmonary artery catheter insertion. In: Sprung CL, ed. *The pulmonary artery catheter: methodology and clinical applications.* Baltimore: University Park Press; 1983:21–72.
5. Sedlock S. Interpretation of hemodynamic pressures and recognition of complications. *Critical Care Nurse.* 1980;Nov–Dec:39–54.
6. Edwards Laboratories. The Swan-Ganz flow-directed thermodilution catheter (package insert). Santa Ana, CA: Edwards Laboratories.
7. Barash P, Kopriva C. Anesthesia for cardiac surgery. In: Glenn W, ed. *Thoracic and cardiovascular surgery.* Norwalk, CT: Appleton-Century-Crofts; 1983:1076–1090.
8. Barash P, Nardi D, Hammond G, et al. Catheter-induced pulmonary artery perforation: mechanisms, management and modifications. *J Thorac Cardiovasc Surg* 1981;82:5–12.
9. Schuster D, Seeman M. Temporary muscle paralysis for accurate measurement of pulmonary artery occlusion pressure. *Chest* 1983;84:593–597.
10. Eaton R, Taxman R, Avioli L. Cardiovascular evaluation of patients treated with PEEP. *Arch Intern Med* 1983;143:1958–1961.
11. Gershan J. Effect of positive end-expiratory pressure on pulmonary capillary wedge pressure. *Heart Lung* 1983;12:143–148.
12. Kopf G, Meshkov A, Laks H, et al. Changing patterns in the surgical management of postinfarction ventricular septal rupture. *Am J Surg* 1982;143:465–472.

13. Hansen RM, Viquerat CE, Matthay MA, Wiener-Kronish JP, et. al. Poor correlation between pulmonary arterial wedge pressure and left ventricular end-diastolic volume after coronary artery bypass graft surgery. *Anesthesiology* 1986;64(6):764-770.
14. Alderman E, Branzi A, Sanders W, et al. Evaluation of the pulse-contour method of determining stroke volume in man. *Circulation* 1972;46:546–558.
15. Karp R, Kouchoukos N. Postoperative care of the cardiovascular surgical patient. In: Glenn W, ed. *Thoracic and cardiovascular surgery.* Norwalk, CT: Appleton-Century-Crofts; 1983:1120–1132.
16. Sprung C, Rackow E, Civetta J. Direct measurements and derived calculations using the pulmonary artery catheter. In: Sprung C, ed. *The pulmonary artery catheter: methodology and clinical applications.* Baltimore: University Park Press; 1983:105–140.
17. Weidemann H, Matthay M, and Matthay R. Cardiovascular-pulmonary monitoring in the intensive care unit (part I). *Chest* 1984;84:537–548.
18. Waller JL, Kaplan JA, Bauman DI, Craver JM. Clinical evaluation of a new fiberoptic catheter during cardiac surgery. *Anesth Analg* 1982;61:676–679.
19. Geha A. Postoperative low cardiac output. In: W. Glenn, ed. *Thoracic and cardiovascular surgery.* Norwalk, CT: Appleton-Century-Crofts; 1983:1133–1146.
20. Boerboom LE, Kinney TE, Olinger GN, Hoffman RG. Validity of cardiac output measurement by the thermodilution method in the presence of acute tricuspid regurgitation. *J Thorac Cardiovasc Surg* 1993;106:636–642.
21. Grondelle A, Ditchey R, Groves B, Wagner W Jr, Reeves J. Thermodilution method overestimates low cardiac output in humans. *Am J Physiol* 1983;245:4690–4692.
22. Elkayan U, Berkley R, Azen S, Weber L, Geva B, Henry W. Cardiac output by thermodilution technique: effect of injectate's volume and temperature on accuracy and reproducibility in the critically ill patient. *Chest* 1983;84:418–422.

SUGGESTED FURTHER READING

Buchbinder N, Ganz W. Hemodynamic monitoring: invasive techniques. *Anesthesiology* 1976;45:146–155.

A brief, succinct discussion of the utility of the Swan-Ganz catheter by one of its originators.

Sprung C. *The pulmonary artery catheter: methodology and clinical applications.* Baltimore: University Park Press; 1983.

A short text devoted to the Swan-Ganz catheter. Recommended for the reader with a special interest in ICU care.

6 Hemodynamic Management

Many factors impair myocardial performance during critical cardiac illness or following cardiac surgery. Acute myocardial infarction obviously destroys cardiac muscle and, accordingly, diminishes pump function. Long-standing valvular or ischemic cardiac disease causes irreparable myocardial damage, irreversible by even the best surgical procedure. Cardiopulmonary bypass and valvular or coronary artery surgery are associated with significant postoperative myocardial depression. Myocardial function improves with every passing hour following cardiac surgery, but several days are usually required before optimization. A given operative procedure may leave certain cardiac defects untreated. For example, mild valvular lesions may be tolerated and valve replacement not performed during a cardiac procedure for another purpose, or a given area of myocardium may prove not amenable to revascularization. Also, metabolic abnormalities abound following cardiac surgery. For all these reasons, myocardial performance may suffer postoperatively. The house officer must be familiar in depth with the optimization of myocardial performance in the setting of acute myocardial infarction and in the postoperative setting. Data obtained via the monitoring techniques discussed in the last chapter form the basis for hemodynamic decisions.

Not only coronary care unit patients and postoperative cardiac surgical patients, but also those in the general surgical intensive care unit may show impaired myocardial performance, as following major abdominal or vascular surgery or from trauma or sepsis. The principles to be enumerated for the cardiac and postoperative cardiac patient apply equally well to optimizing myocardial performance in the acutely ill general surgical patient.

DETERMINANTS OF CARDIAC OUTPUT

Before addressing hemodynamic manipulation, it is useful to examine the clinical factors that influence cardiac output. These are as follows (Fig. 6.1):

81

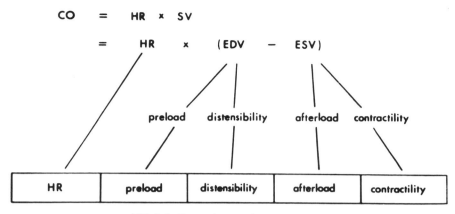

FIG. 6.1. Determinants of cardiac output.

Cardiac output (CO) is the product of heart rate (HR) and stroke volume (SV). That is, if the heart beats 80 times per minute and ejects 60 ml with each beat, it will pump 80 × 60 ml, or 4,800 ml of blood per minute.

Stroke volume is the difference between the ventricular volume at end-diastole (EDV) and the ventricular volume at end-systole (ESV)—that is, the difference between the volume in the ventricle before it beats and the volume remaining after the beat:

$$CO = HR \times SV = HR \times (EDV - ESV)$$

Two factors determine EDV and two factors determine ESV. Those determining EDV, or filling of the ventricle, are **preload** and **ventricular distensibility**. *Preload* represents the pressure driving blood into the ventricle in diastole. The greater the volume in the vascular tree, the greater the driving pressure. *Ventricular distensibility* refers to the degree to which the ventricle can stretch to accommodate volume. A chronically hypertrophied or scarred ventricle may have poor distensibility. The higher the preload and the more distensible the ventricle, the greater will be the EDV.

The factors that determine ESV are **ventricular contractility** and **afterload**. *Ventricular contractility* refers to the "in-shapeness" of the ventricle, that is, the strength of its contraction compared to other conditions or other ventricles. Afterload represents the resistance in the aorta against which the ventricle must pump. A higher systemic blood pressure presents a higher afterload to the ventricle. The greater the contractility and the lower the afterload, the lower will be the ESV; the lower the ESV, the more blood ejected.

Thus the five factors bearing on cardiac output are the following:

1. Heart rate.
2. Preload.
3. Ventricular distensibility.

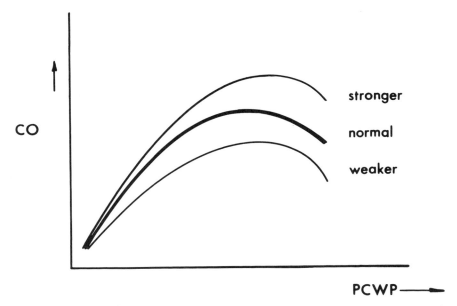

FIG. 6.2. The Frank-Starling mechanism and ventricular function curves. Cardiac output is plotted against PCWP.

4. Contractility.
5. Afterload.

These are the factors that the house officer needs to manipulate in order to optimize CO (1).

The well-known Frank-Starling mechanism and ventricular function curves deserve mention (Fig. 6.2). As the house officer will recall from physiology, the Frank-Starling law states that the larger the diastolic volume of the heart, the more blood the ventricle will pump. In technical terms, stroke volume rises with rising EDV. As will be recalled, this relationship reaches a plateau when ventricular filling becomes excessive. Beyond this point, further increase in filling does not increase CO. If the ventricle is filled significantly beyond the plateau, CO may fall as the ventricle is made to fail from volume overload. Thus for all states of contractility, there is a point on the plateau of the curve at which increasing filling pressure will no longer increase CO.

A strong ventricle will have a curve above and to the left of normal on the CO–PCWP plot. (PCWP is pulmonary capillary wedge pressure.) That is, this ventricle will pump more, at lower filling pressures. A weak ventricle will have a curve below and to the right of normal on the CO–PCWP plot. That is, a weak ventricle will pump less, at higher filling pressures, than a normal one. Stated in another way, the function plateau is reached at a lower level of CO and at higher levels of filling pressure in the impaired than in the normal heart.

CARDIAC OUTPUT MANIPULATION

If CO is found inadequate, remedial measures must be taken. We will now consider how CO can be optimized by adjusting the determinants discussed earlier. Although the major factors determining CO are intimately interrelated, we will examine each separately from the point of view of evaluation and intervention.

Heart Rate

In general, to optimize CO, heart rate must usually be adjusted to the range of 80–110/min. Slower rates are clearly deleterious for ICU patients because CO is determined by rate. We shall explain later why faster rates may be deleterious.

Treatment of bradycardias and of tachycardias has been covered in Chapters 2 and 3. The principles elucidated in those chapters can be applied to obtain rates in the optimal range.

Occasionally, a continuous infusion β-agonist will be selected to increase rate to the upper portion of the optimal range. Dopamine and isoproterenol are often used for this purpose. Use of continuous infusion agents is covered in the next chapter.

One point deserves further elaboration. The house officer may wonder why rates higher than 110/min are not recommended for the ICU patient. Certainly a healthy athlete can continue to increase cardiac output at rates well above 110/min. Two factors compromise the sick or operated heart at higher rates: (1) the time for ventricular filling in diastole falls, and the poorly compliant heart may not fill adequately, and (2) myocardial perfusion suffers, because oxygen demand rises with increasing rate, but diastolic filling time for coronary flow (hence oxygen supply) falls. For these reasons, higher rates are usually detrimental in the ICU patient.

Preload

Adjusting preload is the major intervention required most commonly of the house officer in the care of the patient with coronary ischemia or the postoperative cardiac surgical patient.

As discussed earlier, CO rises as preload is increased—until the optimal preload on the Starling curve is exceeded. By and large, **house officers may on their own initiative raise PCWP to 18–20 mm Hg to optimize CO.** Filling pressures in this range will not overdistend either a normally contractile or a severely diseased heart. An important point deserves emphasis: **It is not necessary to increase filling pressures to this range if a satisfactory CO is achieved at lower filling pressures.** Stated another way, the optimal volume status is that with the lowest filling pressures consistent with a good CO—output being judged not only by computer but by all the criteria discussed in the previous chapter. An efficient heart—for example, that in a young patient without valvular heart disease or prior infarction who undergoes uncomplicated coronary bypass—may be able to pump very well at PCWPs of 10–15 mm Hg. The one very important advantage of running patients as "dry" as possible is that the lungs benefit. With lower filling pressures, the balance of forces across the pulmonary capillary membrane is more in favor of keeping fluid inside the capillary lumen and out of the interstitium, thus improving oxygenation. This is especially important because total body water is always increased after major cardiac surgery and nearly always increased in ICU patients in general.

If CO, as judged by all the preceding criteria, is still seriously inadequate despite achieving a reasonable heart rate and raising PCWP to 18–20 mm Hg, the house officer should seek consultation in further management. Other parameters may need to be manipulated. The experienced clinician will ensure that the other factors (rate, contractility, afterload) are optimized and then proceed further to optimize preload. For the sick heart—especially one that has withstood the insult of major prior infarctions or chronic valvular heart disease, or one that has undergone an especially complex, lengthy, or complicated open-heart procedure—filling pressures higher than 18–20 mm Hg may be required. The preoperative hemodynamics serve as a good guide to postoperative management. The previously described "sick" heart may have functioned at a PCWP of 24 or 28 mm Hg preoperatively. Similarly high pressures may be required postoperatively. The filling pressures required to come off cardiopulmonary bypass during cardiac surgery provide an additional guide. If higher-than-normal pressures were required to come off bypass, chances are that high pressures will be required in the ICU as well.

The experienced clinician in such a setting will judiciously administer fluid to raise filling pressures slowly beyond 20 mm Hg. He or she will monitor cardiac performance closely at these higher pressures, in essence determining the Starling curve for that particular heart. The clinician will carefully avoid overdistending the heart by ceasing volume administration as soon as it becomes apparent that CO is not increasing with added volume. **Overdistention of the postoperative heart is very dangerous.** Laplace's law states that wall tension is proportional to pressure and diameter. Thus wall tension increases as the ventricle is filled further. Wall tension is known to be a major determinant of myocardial oxygen consumption. Thus as the ventricle is distended, myocardial oxygen demand increases. At the same time, however, myocardial oxygen supply decreases, because coronary blood flow is impeded by the elevated left ventricular end-diastolic pressure. The net result is a decrease in the oxygen supply–demand ratio, leading to myocardial ischemia, with its potent negative inotropic effect. The situation may become irretrievable when this occurs, and cardiac arrest may ensue. This is the reason the house officer must seek consultation before raising PCWP above 18–20 mm Hg.

If, under the guidance of an experienced clinician, PCWP is raised to 25 mm Hg and CO is still inadequate, this is a grave sign. Very few hearts require filling pressures higher than this. Chances of recovery from such a state are not great.

If volume excess occurs for any reason, with filling pressures higher than optimal, various pharmacologic vasodilators are available that can lower filling pressures acutely. These are discussed in the next chapter.

Ventricular Distensibility

Ventricular distensibility is the factor in the CO equation over which one has the least control. Distensibility is largely determined by the long-term history of the ventricle. Scarring or hypertrophy from chronic valvular heart disease or hypertension or ischemic infarction will make the ventricle stiff. Such a ventricle will not fill well at normal preload. There is usually no way that this factor can be manipulated or ameliorated acutely or in the postoperative setting. (The one common exception is cardiac tamponade following open-heart surgery; in this instance, relief of tamponade can restore ventricular distensibility.) Some amelioration in ventricular distensibility can be seen over weeks to months after correction of valvular heart disease, especially in aortic stenosis with left ventricular hypertrophy.

Contractility

If CO is inadequate at normal filling pressures, chances are the contractile strength of the heart is inadequate. Under these circumstances, it is appropriate to use an inotropic agent. Again, this is a determination that should not be made by the house officer alone; consultation should be obtained. Inotropic agents are all dangerous. The need to use an inotrope unexpectedly may indicate a major problem— such as cardiac tamponade, myocardial infarction, or valvular prosthetic malfunction—that only the experienced clinician may recognize. Details regarding selection and use of inotropic agents will be discussed in the next chapter.

Again, requirements for coming off bypass serve as a useful guide. If the surgeon finds it necessary to use inotropic support in coming off bypass, chances are that such support will need to be continued in the ICU.

One additional point deserves emphasis. **Acidosis severely depresses contractility, even in the normal heart.** Respiratory or metabolic acidosis must be corrected. Even the response to potent inotropes will be blunted in an acidotic milieu.

Afterload

Afterload, or systemic vascular resistance, can be calculated from the Ohm's law relationship discussed in Chapter 5:

$$\Delta P = CO \times SVR, \text{ or}$$
$$SVR = \Delta P/CO, \text{ or}$$
$$SVR = [BP \text{ (mean)} - RA \text{ (mean)}]/CO$$

Note: ΔP signifies the change in pressure across a vascular bed, in this case, the systemic vasculature. SVR is systemic vascular resistance. CO is cardiac output. BP (mean) is mean arterial blood pressure. RA (mean) is mean right aterial pressure.

Multiplying this value by 80 gives a result in dyne $\times$ sec $\times$ cm^{-5}. The normal range for SVR is 900–1,400.

Afterload manipulation is predicated on the principle that by decreasing arterial pressure in the aorta, it becomes easier for the ventricle to eject blood, thereby increasing CO. This is not without its price, because if aortic pressure is dropped significantly, coronary or other end-organ perfusion (to the brain, intestine, or kidneys) may suffer, especially if the arterial bed to a particular end organ has a fixed stenotic lesion.

The house officer may on his or her own initiative adjust afterload to keep arterial blood pressure at 100–140 mm Hg systolic. Alternatively, mean blood pressure may be adjusted; 70 mm Hg represents the lower acceptable limit (2). In the early postoperative period, one likes to keep arterial pressure below 140 mm Hg to prevent bleeding (see Chapter 10). This goes hand in hand with afterload reduction to improve cardiac function. By and large, house officers should not on their own initiative drop blood pressure below 100 mm Hg systolic for purposes of afterload reduction. This may be necessary in selected cases but should be carried out only after consultation with an experienced clinician. The clinician will carefully assess hemodynamics and risk of end-organ hypoperfusion for that particular patient.

Afterload reduction may be especially helpful in three particular lesions: aortic regurgitation, mitral regurgitation, and ventricular septal defect. In aortic regurgitation, lowering arterial pressure will decrease diastolic backflow across the abnormal valve into the ventricle. In mitral regurgitation, decreasing aortic pressure will decrease peak systolic ventricular pressure commensurately and decrease the fraction of blood regurgitating across the abnormal mitral valve into the left atrium. In ventricular septal defect, for the same reasons, left-to-right ventricular flow during systole is decreased. Ideally, major lesions of this type will be corrected surgically.

Vasodilator Therapy

Vasodilator therapy for cardiac pump failure has come into use relatively recently. The vasodilator agents discussed in the next chapter can be extremely useful in pump failure because of their synergistic effect on preload and afterload. The arterial vasodilator effect decreases afterload, allowing the heart to eject blood more easily. Although the venous vasodilator effect reduces preload, this does not reduce CO appreciably in the failing heart, which is operating on a depressed and flat Frank-Starling relation. The resulting enhancement of the myocardial oxygen supply–demand ratio improves myocardial contractility, further increasing CO.

These principles allow the house officer reliably to assess and to optimize CO. As has been seen, this is done largely by manipulating **rate, preload, contractility, and afterload**.

Mechanical assistance with the intra-aortic balloon pump represents another major modality available for augmentation of cardiac output and myocardial performance. Determining that balloon counterpulsation is required, and inserting the device, should be performed only by the experienced clinician. The intra-aortic balloon pump is covered specifically in Chapter 8.

PATTERNS OF FLUID BALANCE

Cardiopulmonary bypass represents a controlled state of shock. Blood pressure during bypass is usually 40–70 mm Hg. Flow during bypass is nonpulsatile. Effective cardiac index during cardiopulmonary bypass is rarely more than 2.2 liters/min/m². Studies have shown that cell membrane function is disturbed by shock states, so that cells swell diffusely throughout the body (3–5). Under such circumstances, massive volume replacement is required to maintain intravascular volume. The house officer will notice the pattern that, over the 24 h during and after surgery, the cardiac surgical patient often will require several liters of fluid to maintain filling pressures. Much of the house officer's attention during this period is devoted to keeping up with this volume requirement.

The house officer often needs assistance in deciding which fluid to give when volume is necessary. No definitive scientific evidence exists on many aspects of this controversial question. Practices vary from center to center. We practice the following:

- If the hematocrit is less than desired, we give blood, as packed cells. Previously, we kept hematocrit at 30% or greater. In recent years, to avoid transmission of infectious agents, we have allowed hematocrit to drift to 26% or even lower in young, healthy patients without end-organ vascular disease or low cardiac output. (In the presence of end-organ vascular disease or low cardiac output, we still transfuse to 30% hematocrit to maximize oxygen carrying capacity.) Years of experience with hemodilution for cardiopulmonary bypass have shown that low hematocrits are well tolerated, probably because lowered viscosity improves flow and compensates for lowered oxygen-carrying capacity (6).
- If the hematocrit is greater than the criterion level, we give nonblood fluid. We use 5% albumin in D5 1/2NS or hetastarch. Five hundred milliliters given over 1–2 h is a safe volume and rate for an adult. We feel that the colloid of the albumin or hetastarch may help to keep the administered fluid in the vascular tree (7). This has not been demonstrated unequivocally by experimental data, and electrolyte solution alone may suffice.

A common pattern is to give 1 or 2 liters of fluid quickly after arrival of the postcardiac surgical patient in the ICU, and one or two additional liters in 500-ml aliquots at intervals over the first night.

It is uncommon to need to transfuse fluid beyond 24–36 h after surgery. By that time, the "shock" effect has been controlled and myocardial function is improving. The extra fluid required perioperatively will usually be mobilized and excreted as urine over the next 5–7 days.

Urine output patterns deserve mention. Different centers use different regimens of pump fluids and drugs. It is quite common to give diuretics—either the osmotic diuretic mannitol or the loop diuretic furosemide (Lasix)—with the pump prime to keep urine flowing briskly through the tubules. **These agents often lead to a brisk obligatory diuresis in the first 4–6 h after arrival in the ICU.** Osmotic diuresis from postoperative hyperglycemia may compound this obligatory loss. **The house officer usually needs to replace at least one-half to three-fourths of this obligatory urine loss to avoid falling behind on volume.**

By the first or second day after surgery, this obligatory loss has terminated and hormonal effects on urine are seen. **The "stress" response to major cardiac surgery includes up to several days of high antidiuretic hormone and aldosterone secretion** (8). Urine volume may be low because of these hormonal factors. **By and large, after the first 24 h, unless cardiac function is obviously abnormal or volume status obviously and seriously low, oliguria is usually hormonally mediated, and diuretics are required to keep urine flowing and to mobilize excess total body salt and water.** We usually use furosemide (Lasix), 40 mg, at intervals as required. **Valve patients, especially, often come to operation with chronic congestive heart failure and fluid retention and routinely require diuretics after the first night whenever urine output falls.**

COMMON PATTERNS IN VALVULAR HEART DISEASE

Each of the four common valvular lesions causes particular types of dysfunction of which the house officer needs to be aware for proper postoperative management. (See Chapter 13 for more detailed review.)

Aortic stenosis causes severe concentric ventricular hypertrophy. Usually, surgery is performed before irreversible ventricular dysfunction occurs. The hypertrophied ventricle is difficult for the surgeon to protect during the ischemic operative time, but if the operation proceeds smoothly, the ventricle usually functions very well postoperatively. With stenosis relieved, the ventricle functions much more effortlessly.

Aortic regurgitation causes some hypertrophy, but predominantly dilatation results. Dilatation may be advanced by the time of surgery. The dilated, thin-walled ventricle may strain or fail after valve replacement.

Mitral stenosis floods the lungs but protects the ventricle. The left ventricle is neither volume nor pressure overloaded; ventricular function is often well preserved. After relief of stenosis, the ventricle sees more volume load than it is used to, but usually the ventricle is capable of coping well.

Mitral regurgitation places a volume overload on the ventricle, leading to dilatation. This dilated ventricle is often weak. Valve replacement in mitral regurgitation takes a load off the lungs, as the regurgitation into the pulmonary venous system with each beat is immediately controlled. However, **valve replacement for mitral regurgitation is unique among the valvular lesions in placing a severe acute load on the left ventricle.** The dilated left ventricle is used to ejecting a good portion of its end-diastolic volume into the low-pressure left atrium during systole. When a competent prosthetic valve is placed, this low-pressure out-flow is immediately closed; the ventricle sees a much-increased afterload, as all stroke volume must be ejected into the high-pressure aorta. Under these circumstances, the dilated, weakened LV may not tolerate the acute strain brought on by valve replacement and may well fail. In recent years, it has become appreciated as well that the division of the papillary muscles inherent in conventional valve replacement weakens the support of the ventricular wall normally provided by the papillary apparatus, further potentiating the tendency to dilatation and left ventricular failure (9).

REFERENCES

1. Geha A. Postoperative low cardiac output. In: Glenn W, Baue AE, Geha AS, et al, eds. *Thoracic and cardiovascular surgery*, 4th ed. Norwalk, CT: Appleton-Century-Crofts; 1983:1133–1146.
2. Guyton A. *Textbook of medical physiology*, 6th ed. Philadelphia: WB Saunders; 1981.
3. Matthews R, Douglas G. Sulphur-35 measurement of functional and total extracellular fluid in dogs in hemorrhagic shock. *Surg Forum* 1969;20:35.
4. Cunningham J Jr, Shires G, Wagner Y. Cellular transport defects in hemorrhagic shock. *Surgery* 1971;70:215-222.
5. Rutherford R. The pathophysiology of trauma and shock. In: Ballinger W, Rutherford R, Zuidema G, eds. *The management of trauma*. Philadelphia: WB Saunders; 1973:24–69.
6. Lewis D. Resuscitation from shock and trauma—general principles. In: Condon R, Nyhus L, eds. *Manual of surgical therapeutics*, 4th ed. Boston: Little, Brown; 1978:1–11.
7. Virgilio R, Rice C, Smith D, et al. Crystalloid vs. colloid resuscitation: is one better? *Surgery* 1979;85:129–139.
8. Geha, A. Acute renal failure in cardiovascular and other surgical patients. *Surg Clin North Am* 1980;60(5):1151-1166.
9. David T, Komede M, Pollick C, Burns RJ. Mitral valve annuloplasty: The effect of the type on left ventricular function. *Ann Thorac Surg* 1989;47: 524-528.

7 Continuous Infusion Agents

This chapter focuses on those agents that, because of their potency, must be given by carefully controlled continuous infusion in critically ill patients. Each ICU has special drug delivery infusion pumps that are used for this purpose. These powerful agents fall into two general categories: (1) inotropes, which are used to increase the strength of cardiac contraction and often to raise blood pressure (BP), and (2) afterload-reducing agents, which are used to decrease systemic vascular resistance and to lower BP.

INOTROPES

There are many settings in which the strength of cardiac contraction is inadequate; this inadequacy is manifested as low BP or inadequate cardiac output (CO) in the face of adequate preload (normal to high pulmonary capillary wedge pressure; see Chapter 6). This may occur in the coronary care unit following acute myocardial infarction with loss or impairment of significant portions of the left ventricle, in cases of decompensated valvular heart disease, or in the general surgical ICU in very sick patients whose overall septic or traumatic states impair myocardial function. Most commonly, inadequate strength of cardiac contraction is seen in the cardiac ICU following major cardiac surgery using cardiopulmonary bypass.

The heart subjected to major surgery on cardiopulmonary bypass is often very sick. Prior infarcts may have affected large portions of the left ventricle. Acute infarction or ischemia may impair additional muscle. Long-standing valvular heart disease, with pressure or volume overload of the left ventricle, may chronically impair myocardial contractility. Above and beyond the impairment that predates surgery, the operation itself further hampers myocardial function. Most procedures involve a period of time during which the aorta is cross-clamped. During this period, the myocardium is deprived of blood supply. Although modern cardioplegic techniques have greatly improved myocardial preservation during this period, there is no doubt that **the heart that has just come off cardiopulmonary bypass suffers impaired contractility**. Myocardial function will improve minute by minute and hour by hour, especially if appropriate revascularization and valve repair or replacement procedures have been successfully carried out. By 1 or 2 days postoperatively, most of the myocardial depression of surgery will have resolved. From that point on, the heart can "enjoy" and benefit from its newfound blood supply or newly competent valves.

It is common for the heart to require inotropic support following major cardiac procedures on cardiopulmonary bypass. This may manifest in a number of ways. Myocardial function may be inadequate to allow termination of cardiopulmonary bypass. In this case, blood pressure is inadequate despite adequate filling of the heart. In such a case, the surgeon will usually resume bypass, institute inotropic support, and attempt once again to terminate bypass. Often, with inotropic support in effect, the heart can be weaned successfully from cardiopulmonary bypass. In other cases the heart can be successfully weaned from cardiopulmonary bypass without inotropes, but cardiac action is sluggish or CO is low. Again, inotropic support is instituted in such circumstances. The house officer should be aware that **the surgeon generally prefers to institute inotropic support rather than to give volume to the point of overfilling and overdistending the heart that has just come off cardiopulmonary bypass**. The heart just off bypass is very vulnerable; distention increases wall tension and myocardial workload and oxygen demand; the volume-overloaded heart may not be able to cope and may fail acutely or fibrillate.

In other patients, myocardial performance in the operating room may appear satisfactory; at some time following return to the ICU, however, CO may become inadequate. This may manifest as hypotension, poor peripheral perfusion, poor urine output, poor mixed venous O_2, poor measured CO, and so on, as discussed in Chapter 6.

In any of these circumstances, in the coronary care unit, the general surgical ICU, or the cardiac surgical ICU, a choice of inotropic agent must be made. **Five continuous infusion catecholamines are in common clinical use as inotropic agents: norepinephrine, epinephrine, isoproterenol, dopamine, and dobutamine.** (Table 7.1) (1–7). **One noncatecholamine—amrinone—is also commonly used for inotropic support. Milrinone is a new agent in the same category as amrinone, which is gaining popularity.**

The catecholamine agents differ in the balance of α- and β-effects generated. **Pure α-agonists cause predominantly peripheral vasoconstriction without primary cardiac enhancement. β-agonists increase heart rate and myocardial contractility; they also often cause peripheral vasodilatation.** Table 7.1 indicates the relative α-and β-activity of each agent. At one extreme is norepinephrine, which has predominantly α-activity as well as some β-agonism. At the other extreme is isoproterenol, which has almost exclusively β-activity; isoproterenol is **the** β-agonist. The other agents have mixed effects. Epinephrine has both α- and β-activity. For dopamine and dobutamine, α- and β-agonism varies with dosage range (see later). For a given patient, one of these drugs may provide the most appropriate balance of α- and β-activity. **In general, α-agonists, although they raise blood pressure, are frowned**

Table 7.1. *Inotropic agents in common use*

Generic name (Trade name)	Activity	Dilution	Dose range	Comments
Norepinephrine (Levophed)	$\alpha > \beta$	2 mg/250 ml (8 µg/ml)	0.02 -0.2 µg/kg/min	Rarely useful—peripheral vascoconstriction overshadows positive inotropism
Epinephrine (Adrenalin)	α and β	1 mg/250 ml (4 µg/ml)	0.01-0.1 µg/kg/min	Useful agent
Dopamine (Inotropin)	α and β	200 mg/250 ml (800 µg/ml)	1-30 µg/kg/min	Useful agent Dose-related pattern of effect: 1-2 µg/kg/min—renal vasodilation 2-10 µg/kg/min—β-agonism 10-15 µg/kg/min— α- and β-agonism >15 µg/kg/min—α-agonism Compared to more potent agents: Less tachycardic effect Less arrhythmogenicity
Dobutamine (Dobutrex)	α and β	250 mg/250 ml (1,000 µg/ml)	1-30 µg/kg/min	Useful agent No specific renal vasodilatory effect Little tachycardic effect
Isoproterenol (Isuprel)	β	1 mg/250 ml (1,000 µg/ml)	0.01 - 0.1 µg/kg/min	Useful agent—*the* β-agonist
Milrinone (Primacor)	NA	1 mg/ml	0.375 - 0.75 µg/kg/min	Loading dose 50 µg/kg
Amrinone (Inocor)	NA	200 mg/250 ml (800 µcg/ml)	5 - 40 µcg/kg/min	Non-catecholamine Loading dose 1 - 2 mg/kg

upon, because the increased afterload increases myocardial workload and oxygen consumption and often decreases CO despite the increased BP.

The house officer will notice from Table 7.1 that the listed agents fall into two categories of potency. Norepinephrine, epinephrine, and isoproterenol are potent agents, active in doses on the order of hundredths of a microgram per kilogram per minute. Dopamine and dobutamine are less potent agents, requiring microgram-per-kilogram doses about 100 times greater than the more potent agents. At our center, **we prefer the potent agents for patients who have serious difficulties after cardiopulmonary bypass; the less potent agents are preferred for patients who merely require some inotropism in the ICU to optimize hemodynamics.** Usage patterns vary greatly from center to center. Many centers do use dopamine or dobutamine, in high-dosage ranges, for patients seriously ill in the operating room; this usage pattern can also be effective.

Table 7.1 includes recommended dilutions for these potent agents. These dilutions each represent "one amp" (one commercial ampule of drug) per 250-ml bag of solution. With these dilutions, infusion rates of 20–60 ml/h will give dosages in the middle of the recommended ranges for most adults. Standard dilutions vary from center to center; any dilution can be used as long as the rate of administration is appropriately adjusted.

The house officer should be aware that an individual patient may respond to one inotropic agent but not to another. If one agent, even a potent one, fails to maintain BP or CO, a switch to another agent should be made. All experienced cardiac surgeons can recall thinking all to be lost in a particular case only to see a dramatic and sustained response with a change to another, "last-ditch" inotrope. On certain occasions, the experienced clinician will even administer concomitantly two or more different inotropic agents.

Norepinephrine (Levophed)

Norepinephrine is a potent catecholamine with both α- and β-activity. Because α-activity usually predominates, norepinephrine is not currently thought to be beneficial to most patients; its peripheral vasoconstriction overshadows its inotropism. Although blood pressure will increase, this is at the expense of increased afterload on the heart; cardiac output may actually decrease. Nevertheless, some patients whose blood pressure cannot be maintained by other drugs can be salvaged by the use of norepinephrine.

Norepinephrine can at times be useful to improve coronary perfusion by raising central aortic pressure. At times, this may interrupt a vicious cycle of inadequate cardiac function, hypotension, decreased coronary flow, and further impairment of cardiac function. This paradigm underlies the use of norepinephrine in cardiac tamponade (see Chapter 16) and after cardiac arrest (see Chapter 10).

Norepinephrine is specifically indicated in those patients with hypotension from decreased systemic vascular resistance (with preserved CO). This can be seen in sepsis and following severe neurologic events. The dysfunction is not primarily cardiac in this setting.

Some surgeons use a so-called Canadian cocktail for patients who cannot be weaned from cardiopulmonary bypass. This cocktail is made by combining norepinephrine with the potent vasodilator phentolamine (Regitine) in a 4:5 ratio by milligram (6). The phentolamine completely counteracts norepinephrine's peripheral vasoconstriction, leaving strong, unopposed inotropism. This cocktail is indeed a potent and effective inotrope.

Epinephrine (Adrenalin)

Epinephrine is a potent catecholamine with both α- and β-activity. Unlike the vasoconstriction resulting from norepinephrine, that from epinephrine does not outshine inotropism. The balance of actions is more suitable with this drug for primary cardiac dysfunction, especially when any of the afterload-reducing agents discussed later is administered concomitantly. Epinephrine is often the first agent selected for the patient who needs help coming off cardiopulmonary bypass or who shows severely inadequate CO in the ICU.

Isoproterenol (Isuprel)

Isoproterenol has almost pure β-activity (1). For this reason, it is considered by many the inotrope of choice for patients who cannot be weaned from cardiopulmonary bypass or who manifest severely low CO. Because it has almost no α-activity, isoproterenol may actually **lower** BP, while increasing CO; this may occur because the unopposed β-agonism produces peripheral vasodilatation in addition to inotropism.

Isoproterenol is intensely arrhythmogenic. Serious ventricular arrhythmias are commonly seen with moderate-to-high dose administration.

One major advantage of isoproterenol is that it is the only one of the potent inotropes that decreases pulmonary vascular resistance. This aspect of the action of isoproterenol is particularly useful in patients with chronic pulmonary hypertension (especially mitral valve patients) and in patients with acute right ventricular failure.

Dopamine (Inotropin)

Dopamine is a very useful agent from the category of less potent inotropes. The difference in potency is partially compensated by a 100-fold increase in concentration of the solution prepared (see Table 7.1).

The balance of α- and β-effects with dopamine varies with the rate of administration. At infusion rates of 1–2 μg/kg/min, specific renal vasodilatation predominates. At 2–10 μg/kg/min, β-activity predominates above α-activity. At greater than 10 μg/kg/min, α-activity increases, and above 15 μg/kg/min α-activity predominates.

Many surgeons find dopamine a nearly ideal agent in the 5- to 10-μg/kg/min range of administration. This agent provides significant augmentation of contractility. Less tachycardia and less arrhythmogenicity are seen than with epinephrine or isoproterenol. For these reasons, at some centers dopamine is the agent of choice for low-output states or even for weaning from cardiopulmonary bypass. Nonetheless, in certain cases, despite higher concentrations, dopamine just does not provide the strength of effect that epinephrine or isoproterenol does.

Although dopamine is known to dilate the renal vasculature, the house officer often overestimates the significance of this effect. Dopamine has never been shown to alter the course of acute tubular necrosis in humans (7).

Dobutamine (Dobutrex)

Dobutamine is another useful agent from the category of less potent inotropes. Overall dosages are similar to those for dopamine. Unlike dopamine, dobutamine has no specific renal vasodilating effect. In its favor, dobutamine causes even less tachycardia and is less arrhythmogenic than dopamine. Dobutamine produces a fall in systemic vascular resistance, even in the high-dosage range.

Amrinone (Inocor)

Amrinone is a relatively recently introduced inotropic agent that belongs to a completely different category of drugs than the agents discussed up to this point. The other agents discussed earlier all stimulate α- and/or β-receptors in cardiac muscle and blood vessels. Amrinone belongs to a class of agents that inhibit phosphodiesterase (thus the name of the category, *phosphodiesterase inhibitors*, or PDE inhibitors). Phosphodiesterase inhibition increases cyclic AMP (adenosine monophosphate) levels, improving the contractile mechanism of cardiac muscle. It is important to emphasize that this mechanism of action is entirely different from that of the catecholamines. (The loading dose is 1–2 mg/kg; the maintenance dose is 2–20 µg/kg/min.)

Amrinone has been found to be a useful agent for congestive heart failure and for postoperative low cardiac output (8). The house officer will find this agent useful in both the coronary care unit and the postoperative cardiac intensive care unit. Amrinone increases cardiac output. Because the mechanism of increase in cardiac output does not involve catecholamine stimulation, the cardiac output increases without increase in heart rate. Because the heart rate does not increase, myocardial oxygen demand does not increase. For similar reasons, amrinone is not arrhythmogenic. Also, unlike most catecholamines, amrinone decreases systemic vascular resistance. This effect further helps to increase cardiac output and to decrease myocardial oxygen demand. Thus amrinone has the advantages of increasing cardiac output without increasing heart rate or myocardial oxygen demand.

An additional advantage of amrinone is its ability to decrease pulmonary vascular resistance. This can be of particular importance in patients with mitral valve disease and increased pulmonary vascular resistance on that basis. The ability to decrease pulmonary vascular resistance makes amrinone specifically useful in patients with right ventricular failure, as after right ventricular infarction or pulmonary embolism.

Yet an additional advantage of amrinone is a synergistic effect when combined with catecholamine treatment. By virtue of their different mechanisms of action, amrinone and catecholamines, when used together, produce an improvement in cardiac performance greater than that of either drug used alone. It is very common, in the setting of seriously low cardiac output following cardiac surgery, for the house officer to find the patient on both amrinone and a powerful catecholamine.

Because of the unique advantages described above, amrinone has, in a short time, become a very widely used myocardial stimulant. Some authors have even advocated prophylactic treatment with a bolus of amrinone before initiating cardiopulmonary bypass in high-risk candidates, so that a level of drug will already be on board by the completion of the open-heart procedure.

Milrinone is a relatively recently introduced PDE-III inhibitor that is 10 to 30 times more potent than amrinone. Doses are correspondingly smaller, which may reduce side effects. Thrombocytopenia is not a problem with milrinone. Milrinone's shorter half-life may represent an advantage in the acute care setting. The loading dose is 50 µg/kg infused over 10 minutes and the recommended continuous infusion is 0.375–0.76 µg/Kg/min.

AFTERLOAD-REDUCING AGENTS

Pharmacologic intervention to reduce afterload is required most commonly for the severe hypertension that so often follows cardiac surgery. Many factors may enter into producing this postoperative hypertension. Catecholamine and renin-angiotensin excess may be involved. Generalized hypothermia and concomitant vasoconstriction increase afterload and cause hypertension (9). Whatever the cause, hypertension promotes bleeding (see Chapter 15) and reduces CO (see Chapter 6). Postoperative hypertension must always be corrected, and it is the afterload-reducing agents discussed in this section that are used for that purpose.

As discussed in Chapter 6, afterload reduction is also used, even in normotensive patients, to increase CO in low-output states associated with congestive failure and to minimize the impact of the mechanical lesions of acute ventricular septal defect and acute mitral regurgitation. The agents to be discussed are useful in these settings as well.

Three drugs are used commonly by continuous infusion in the intensive care setting to reduce blood pressure and afterload: sodium nitroprusside, trimethaphan, and nitroglycerin (Table 7.2) (10). These agents are so potent that beat-to-beat monitoring of arterial pressure by arterial line is a necessity for their use.

Table 7.2 *Afterload-reducing agents used by continuous infusion*

Generic Name (Trade Name)	Arterial or Venous Predominance	Dilution	Dose Range	Toxicity	Comments
Sodium nitropruside (Nipride)	Arterial	100 mg/250 ml	1-10 µg/kg/min	Cyanide intoxication Increased intrapulmonary shunting	Mainstay agent Degraded by light
Trimethaphan (Arfonad)	Arterial	500 mg/250 ml	1-6 mg/min	Negative inotropism	Less immediate effect Tachyphylaxis may occur
Nitroglycerine (TNG)	Venous	200 µg/ml	1-5 µg/kg/min	None	Special beneficial effects on myocardial O_2 supply/demand balance

Sodium Nitroprusside (Nipride)

Nitroprusside is an extremely effective afterload-reducing agent. Almost all patients respond. Nitroprusside acts by a direct effect on both capacitance (venous) and resistance (arterial) vessels (10). Venodilatation reduces blood pressure by way of decreased venous return and decreased CO. This can be compensated by volume repletion. Arteriolar dilatation reduces blood pressure by way of afterload reduction, often with an increase in CO.

Nitroprusside will lower blood pressure within seconds to minutes of administration. Likewise, nitroprusside's effect will dissipate within seconds to minutes of discontinuance. This immediacy of response and predictability make nitroprusside especially appropriate for the postoperative cardiac patient, in whom conditions may change very quickly.

Nitroprusside may be prepared as 100 mg in 250 ml of solution. Accepted chronic infusion rates up to 8 μg/kg/min are safe (10). In our unit, we use up to 10 μg/kg/min overnight following cardiac surgery without problem. This translates to an infusion rate of 100 ml/h for the 70-kg male at the dilution stated. This maximum safe rate of 100 ml/h is easy for the house officer to recall. Nitroprusside is degraded by light exposure, so infusion bags are commonly wrapped in foil or other opaque coverings. The dissolved drug is normally pale brown and turns blue when degraded by light.

The major serious toxicity of nitroprusside is cyanide intoxication. The chemical makeup of nitroprusside includes five cyanide radicals. These can be liberated by metabolism of nitroprusside. It is interesting to note that metabolism is believed to occur mainly with hemoglobin rather than in the liver. Excess dosage must be used for a prolonged period for toxicity to develop. This occurs only rarely. Caution in dosage should be exercised when a patient develops tachyphylaxis—that is, when a patient who previously responded requires more and more drug for an effect to be seen. When toxicity does occur, it may manifest via acidosis (from anaerobic tissue metabolism necessitated by the poisoning of the aerobic cycle by cyanide) and via elevated mixed venous O_2 (from interference in oxygen extraction) (10). Treatment regimens for toxicity have been described (4).

Another possible toxic effect of nitroprusside is an increase in right-to-left shunting with resultant hypoxia (11,12). This is not commonly problematic in clinical practice.

Nitroprusside will become a close friend to the house officer who spends some time in a cardiac intensive care unit.

Trimethaphan (Arfonad)

Trimethaphan also reduces blood pressure by a combination of capacitance and resistance vessel dilatation. This drug is a ganglionic blocker; its dilatory effects stem from blocking of sympathetic efferent signals.

This drug is prepared as 500 mg in 250 ml of solution. The dosage range is 1–6 mg/min.

Trimethaphan can be used very effectively for postoperative blood pressure control. It is, however, a second-line agent behind nitroprusside for a number of reasons. Trimethaphan does not have quite as immediate an onset and termination of effect. Tachyphylaxis is not uncommon with trimethaphan. Also, trimethaphan has some negative inotropic effects (4) that may decrease CO.

Nitroglycerin (TNG)

Nitroglycerin has been used for over 100 years as the mainstay of treatment for angina. Intravenous nitroglycerin is a useful vasodilator for the postoperative open-heart patient, especially following coronary artery bypass grafting, and for the patient in coronary care with active myocardial ischemia (3,4,13). (See Chapter 12.)

Nitroglycerin has more predominant capacitance (venous) vessel effects than does nitroprusside. At doses of nitroglycerin of less than 1 μg/kg/min, venodilatation predominates. At higher doses, some arterial dilatation occurs. As might be expected from this balance of effects, nitroglycerin is a more effective reducer of preload than of afterload. Nonetheless, some measure of blood pressure control can be achieved with nitroglycerin in the postoperative setting.

If nitroglycerin is not as effective in blood pressure control as nitroprusside, why is it used after cardiac surgery? In very basic terms, nitroglycerin is good for the heart with coronary disease. Nitroglycerin exerts a beneficial effect on the oxygen demand–supply ratio by influencing both sets of factors in this ratio. Oxygen demand is decreased, largely by way of reduction in preload, with concomitant reduction in wall tension and energy requirements. This can be accomplished as well by nitroprusside. Unlike nitroprusside, however, nitroglycerin can increase oxygen supply. Nitroglycerin is known to dilate coronary arteries; this effect is demonstrated routinely during coronary angiography. Both large and small coronary arteries, including collateral vessels, are dilated by nitroglycerin. This may increase flow to the vulnerable subendocardial myocardium. Although it is true that fixed anatomic coronary lesions cannot respond to nitroglycerin, the spasm that often superimposes on fixed anatomic lesions may respond dramatically. Collateral flow around a fixed anatomic lesion may be improved as well. Nitroglycerin has been shown to improve ischemic EKG changes during coronary artery bypass surgery (14).

Now why would a postoperative patient still be at risk for ischemia following coronary artery bypass grafting? First, coronary spasm can occur following bypass—at times to a severe extent. Second, it is unusual to achieve total coronary revascularization—that is, to make the patient's coronaries entirely normal. More often than not, small diseased vessels remain. Vessels less than 1.5 mm in diameter are usually not grafted. Also, some milder disease usually persists beyond the major lesions bypassed. Distal disease is especially common in diabetics. The initial period following coronary artery surgery is a critical one (see Chapter 6). The heart needs all the help it can get during this time. Nitroglycerin may provide just that increased margin of coronary blood flow required to keep even the adequately revascularized patient out of trouble during the vulnerable early postoperative period.

Concentrations of nitroglycerin in commercial preparations vary. In our unit, the nitroglycerin comes as 200 μg/ml. Nitroglycerin has no known serious toxicity. Headaches do occur but are not of importance in the heavily sedated patient emerging from cardiac surgery. Accordingly, there is no definite known maximum tolerable dose. Common ranges are 1–4 μg/kg/min. It is unusual to see much additional benefit at doses beyond 4 μg/kg/min.

In our postcardiac surgical unit, we use both nitroglycerin and nitroprusside in many patients. Nitroglycerin is started initially, to gain some measure of blood pressure control and to benefit from its coronary vasodilating properties. The rate of infusion of nitroglycerin is increased to maintain control of hypertension. Once medium-dose ranges of nitroglycerin are reached, nitroprusside is added if required for blood pressure control. In this way, the coronary benefits of nitroglycerin are combined with the potent afterload-reducing properties of nitroprusside. These agents are usually tapered (not abruptly discontinued) the day following surgery, when blood pressure control can safely be liberalized (see Chapter 15).

Bolus Agents

Unlike the afterload-reducing agents discussed thus far, chlorpromazine (Thorazine) and hydralazine (Apresoline) are usually given by bolus injection rather than by continuous infusion. These two additional agents may be useful to the house officer in controlling postoperative hypertension.

Chlorpromazine is used in our unit for the patient who remains hypertensive despite maximal doses of nitroprusside. This scenario is not uncommon. Thorazine produces a prompt vasodilatation and lowering of blood pressure. This more or less "resets" the blood pressure mechanism to a lower absolute value; fine tuning is done by regulating nitroprusside, but now at safe dosage levels.

Chlorpromazine is a potent vasodilator. It can drop BP severely. For this reason, we use it cautiously. We give a 2.5-mg bolus at one time, repeating as necessary every 5–10 min, up to a total of 15 mg. The house officer should have a volume agent (crystalloid, colloid, or blood) available to replete the vascular compartment if BP falls precipitously after chlorpromazine, as this bolus agent cannot be titrated instantaneously, as can the continuous infusion agents discussed earlier.

Chlorpromazine is, of course, a sedative agent, and its overuse can result in worrisome depression of mental status following open-heart surgery. We try to use as little of this agent as possible, just to keep our nitroprusside administration in a safe range.

Hydralazine can be used by the house officer to effect a transition from continuous infusion agents to bolus agents—to "get the patient off drips," in effect. By the first or second day after surgery, vasoconstriction and severe hypertension usually resolve. BP control can be liberalized, as bleeding is no longer likely and the heart is no longer as vulnerable to increased afterload. BP that was maintained at 110–120 mm Hg early after surgery can be liberalized to 140–160 mm Hg. Hydralazine given by bolus can provide this measure of blood pressure control and allow the continuous infusion of nitroprusside to be stopped.

Hydralazine is a potent direct arterial vasodilator. It must be used with caution. Common doses are 10–50 mg IV every 4–6 h. The house officer is advised to start with low doses and and to increase them gradually. The drug can be given in about the same doses orally when the patient begins oral intake. If tachycardia is seen during hydralazine treatment, or as a general response to the postoperative state (see Chapter 2), it is convenient to add a β-blocker (like propranolol). The β-blocker will further facilitate BP control.

Methyldopa (Aldomet), an adrenergic blocking agent, was popular in previous years for BP control following cardiac surgery. This drug can be given as 250–500 mg IV or p.o. every 6 h. Aldomet is quite effective but may take up to 48 h to achieve the reduction in BP. Because of this delay in action, and because hydralazine with propranolol makes such an effective and convenient combination, Aldomet has largely been supplanted at our institution.

Nifedipine, given sublingually at 10–20 mg every 4–6 h, is also an effective bolus agent for blood pressure control.

REFERENCES

1. Innes IR, Nickerson M. Drugs acting on postganglionic adrenergic nerve endings and structures innervated by them (sympathomimetic drugs). In: Goodman L, Gilman A, eds. *The pharmacologic basis of therapeutics.* New York: Macmillan; 1970:478–523.
2. White R. Cardiovascular pharmacology. Part I. In: McIntyre K, Lewis A, eds. *Textbook of advanced cardiac life support.* Dallas: American Heart Association; 1981:VIII-1–VIII-16.
3. McIntyre K. Cardiovascular pharmacology. Part II. In: McIntyre K, Lewis A, eds. *Textbook of advanced cardiac life support.* Dallas: American Heart Association; 1981:IX-1–IX-16.
4. Glass D. Cardiovascular drugs. In: Civetta J, ed. *Intensive care therapeutics.* New York: Appleton-Century-Crofts; 1980:197–261.
5. Zito R. Cardiovascular clinical pharmacology. In: Glenn W, Baue AE, Geha AS, et al, eds. *Thoracic and cardiovascular surgery,* 4th ed. Norwalk, CT: Appleton-Century-Crofts; 1983:1063–1075.
6. Behrendt D, Austen W. *Patient care in cardiac surgery.* Boston: Little, Brown; 1980.
7. Raijfer S, Goldberg L. Sympathomimetic amines in the treatment of shock. In: Shoemaker W, Thompson W, Holbrook P, eds. *Textbook of critical care.* Philadelphia: WB Saunders; 1984.
8. Hines R. Preoperative and postoperative use of inotropes in cardiac surgery. *J Cardiothorac Anesth* (Suppl 5) 1990;4:29–33.
9. Hoar P, Stone J, Faltas A, et al. Hemodynamic and adrenergic responses to anesthesia and operation for myocardial revascularization. *J Thorac Cardiovasc Surg* 1980;80:242–248.
10. Stinson E, Holloway E, Derby R, et al. Comparative hemodynamic responses to chlorpromazine, nitroprusside, nitroglycerin, and trimethaphan immediately after open heart operations. *Circulation* (Suppl) 1975;51/52:26–33.
11. Michenfelder J. Sodium nitroprusside therapy. *Weekly Anesthesiology Update* 1978;2:2–8.
12. Brodie T, Gray R, Swan H, Matloff S. Effect of nitroprusside on arterial oxygenation, intrapulmonic shunts, and oxygen delivery. *Am J Cardiol* 1976;37:123.
13. Purcell J, Holder C. Intravenous nitroglycerin. *Am J Nursing* 1982;82:254–259.
14. Kaplan J, Jones E. Vasodilator therapy during coronary artery surgery. Comparison of nitroglycerin and nitroprusside. *J Thorac Cardiovasc Surg* 1979;77:301–309.

SUGGESTED FURTHER READING

Management of surgical low cardiac output syndrome. Levy JH, Wynands JE, eds. *J Cardiothorac Anesth* (Suppl 5) 1990;4:1–41.

An up-to-date and lucid monograph by experts like Dr. Hines (see Ref. 8), although weighted in favor of the PDE inhibitors.

8 The Intra-aortic Balloon Pump

The house officer is often frightened at the prospect of caring for a patient with an intra-aortic balloon pump (IABP). Yet more and more patients are becoming candidates for intra-aortic balloon counterpulsation (1–4). This chapter will review important basic concepts regarding the balloon pump with which the house officer should be familiar.

PHYSICAL CHARACTERISTICS

The balloon itself is an inflatable plastic device that is positioned in the descending aorta, usually via the common femoral artery. The balloon is attached to a console, which monitors either EKG or arterial pressure. The console triggers the balloon in concert with the EKG or arterial pressure. **The balloon is inflated in diastole and deflated in systole.** (The volume in adults is usually 40 ml.) **This provides systolic unloading and diastolic augmentation** (Fig. 8.1). This is a difficult concept to grasp and requires further elaboration.

PHYSIOLOGIC EFFECTS

Consider the events of the cardiac cycle, starting in diastole just after aortic valve closure, with the IABP functioning. The balloon inflates in the thoracic aorta. This raises the diastolic pressure in the aorta and displaces an additional volume of blood, equal to that of the balloon, from the aorta into runoff organs—a sort of augmentation of cardiac output. One of the organs that benefits most is the heart, as some of the displaced volume passes down the coronary arteries. The increased diastolic pressure in the aorta is especially beneficial because it is during diastole that most coronary flow occurs. During systole, the myocardium is contracting, and the pressure

103

FIG. 8.1. Timing of the IABP. The top trace shows EKG. The second trace marks balloon inflation and deflation. The third trace shows pressure in the balloon itself. The final trace represents intra-arterial blood pressure. (The dotted line represents the arterial pressure curve that would obtain without the IABP; the solid line indicates the curve with IABP.) The cross-hatched areas represent lowering of blood pressure in systole (systolic unloading) and raising of blood pressure in diastole (diastolic augmentation).

exerted on the coronaries by the surrounding myocardium prevents significant coronary flow.

The balloon is maintained inflated by the console until just before systole, when balloon deflation occurs. This lowers systolic pressure in the aorta and makes it easier for the left ventricle to eject its stroke volume. The workload of the left ventricle is diminished.

Thus the IABP is beneficial to the heart because (1) diastolic augmentation improves coronary flow and myocardial oxygen supply, and (2) systolic unloading decreases the workload of the left ventricle and myocardial oxygen demand. The combination of greater coronary flow with less load on the heart can produce a dramatic improvement in myocardial performance.

It is instructive to compare the use of IABP for hypotension and low cardiac output to conventional medical intervention. β-Agonists can increase cardiac output, but at the expense of increased myocardial oxygen consumption. α-Agonists can raise BP, but at the expense of increased afterload and, again, increased myocardial oxygen consumption. Only the IABP can effect amelioration of this circulatory state *without* increased oxygen consumption. As myocardial ischemia is so commonly the cause of the low-output state, this advantage of the IABP may be truly critical.

APPLICATIONS

The IABP is used most commonly in three situations. It can be used following open-heart surgery to assist a weak heart in sustaining the circulation after coming off cardiopulmonary bypass. Another setting of common use is in the preoperative patient in the coronary care unit who continues to have angina despite full treatment with β-blockers, calcium antagonists, and nitrates (usually intravenous nitroglycerin). Because it decreases cardiac workload and increases flow through the diseased coronary vessels, the IABP almost always eliminates even refractory anginal pain. In addition, the IABP may be used to support the failing heart in postmyocardial infarction (cardiogenic) shock.

There are other, less common settings in which the IABP may be used. The mechanical defects of ventricular septal rupture and acute mitral regurgitation may follow myocardial infarction. Both of these life-threatening complications can be ameliorated by the IABP. The systolic unloading decreases peak left ventricular pressures; this, in turn, decreases left-to-right shunting in acute ventricular septal defect and decreases regurgitation into the atrium in acute mitral valve dysfunction. In these settings, the IABP is usually used as an adjunct in the preparation of the patient for surgery for correction of the mechanical defect. In addition, the IABP may be used to protect coronary patients with especially precarious anatomy during induction of anesthesia and the precardiopulmonary bypass period of the coronary bypass operation. Patients with severe left main coronary lesions may require this protection. Use of the IABP for left main disease is becoming less common as monitoring and anesthetic techniques improve. In rare cases, the IABP may be useful in controlling refractory, life-threatening ventricular arrhythmias.

As patients with more advanced left ventricular dysfunction and more complex cardiac disease are submitted to corrective open-heart procedures, an important role is emerging for the IABP for prophylactic peri-operative (pre- and postoperative) support electively around the time of cardiac surgery. It used to be felt that the IABP could be applied in case of inadequate pump function in the operating room at the completion of the open-heart repair. Our group has found the IABP extremely useful as a *prophylactic* measure, especially for coronary bypass in patients with severe preexisting damage and for left ventricular aneurysmectomy (especially aneurysmectomy combined with directed arrhythmia surgery) (5,6).

One major contraindication to use of the IABP is aortic regurgitation. The principles of operation of the IABP enumerated earlier presume a competent aortic valve. Without aortic valve competence, inflation of the balloon in diastole may exacerbate the regurgitation from the aorta to the left ventricle, possibly overwhelming the ventricle.

POSITIONING AND REMOVAL

In its early use, the IABP was placed by a surgical procedure to expose the common femoral artery and anastomose a diverticulum of Dacron or Teflon to the side of the vessel. The balloon was then passed through the diverticulum. Subsequently, the Seldinger technique for passing the IABP has been popularized. With this technique the IABP, which has a central lumen, is passed over a guide wire through a sheath placed into the common femoral artery. The guide wire and sheath can be placed percutaneously. IABP removal can be done closed (with pressure to control the arterial site) or open (with direct repair of the arterial site). A sheathless model of the IABP (which has a tapered, firm tip) is now entering clinical use (Datascope, Montvale, New Jersey); this model is placed directly through the skin over a guide wire into the femoral artery, eliminating the sheath and thus decreasing the overall diameter of the apparatus.

CARE AND COMPLICATIONS

The IABP can result in aortic dissection or vascular perforation during its introduction, especially in a patient with aortoiliac disease. The incidence of these serious, and often fatal, complications has been markedly reduced by the use of a wire-guided central lumen balloon.

The IABP can impair blood flow to the extremity supplied by the femoral artery through which it is introduced (7). This is especially likely when there is associated aortoiliac or femoropopliteal occlusive disease, when the IABP is inadvertently introduced through the superficial femoral artery rather than through the common femoral, or when cardiac output is very low. **The house officer must closely monitor lower-extremity perfusion in the patient with the IABP**, using all traditional criteria (pulses, warmth, color, sensation, motor strength, etc).

The IABP is traumatic to formed blood elements, especially platelets. The house officer must follow platelet counts closely, especially when the IABP has been in place more than 12 or 24 h (8). Falling counts or counts below 40,000 should be called to the attention of senior staff.

The IABP can provide a nidus for intra-arterial thrombosis and embolization. Clot forms on the inflating/deflating balloon membrane itself. Clot is less likely to form when the balloon is firing frequently. If the balloon were not to fire for a significant period of time, thrombosis would be almost certain. For this reason, **we never run the IABP at a rate of less than 1:4** (i.e., one IABP inflation for every four heartbeats) **for any significant period of time.**

The question of anticoagulation of patients with the IABP deserves elaboration. There is much variation in operating principles from center to center. Our operating protocols will be described to serve as a baseline for the house officer.

We do anticoagulate patients who have the IABP placed preoperatively. We do this with heparin by continuous infusion (usually 800–1,000 units/h IV). We stop the heparin several hours preoperatively.

We do not anticoagulate patients who have the IABP in place postoperatively. After cardiac surgery, blood coagulation mechanisms are disturbed. Further, with fresh incisions and suture lines, anticoagulation would not be safe. The IABP is usually withdrawn by the time coagulation normalizes and anticoagulation would be safe. If the IABP were required for a prolonged period of time—say, beyond the second preoperative day—some form of anticoagulation would be considered.

The house officer should understand the process of "timing" the IABP (see Fig. 8.1). Adjustments of timing are necessary with changes in rhythm or rate and can be done by the house officer with an understanding of the process. As mentioned, the IABP may be triggered by the EKG or by the arterial trace; likewise, it can be set according to the electrical events of the EKG or the mechanical events of the arterial pressure monitor. We shall discuss both techniques of setting timing.

The initial setting is done by EKG. **The IABP should be set to inflate at the peak of the T wave**; by this point in the EKG, systole is certain to be complete. **The IABP is set to deflate just before the beginning of the QRS**; in this manner, it will be deflated before any significant mechanical contraction of the ventricle occurs with the next systole. The reader should follow the EKG timing in Fig. 8.1.

Fine tuning can be done by observing the arterial trace. **The IABP-augmented pressure should begin where the dicrotic notch would start.** Inflation is moved forward or backward to achieve this. **The presystolic dip in pressure should be as low as possible.** Deflation can be moved forward or backward to achieve this.

One usually finds that tuning by the dicrotic notch on the arterial trace sets IABP inflation a little more accurately than the peak of the T wave by EKG. On the other hand, setting deflation at the beginning of the QRS rarely requires adjustment based on the arterial trace. To summarize, then

Set inflation to occur at the dicrotic notch of the A-line.
Set deflation to occur just before the QRS of the EKG.

As rate changes or as rhythm varies, the inflate/deflate timing will need to be adjusted. If a paced rhythm becomes necessary, major readjustment of inflation/deflation will be required. In this circumstance, the arterial trace is the best guide. It must be remembered that an improperly timed IABP may well impair cardiac function. This would be the case, for example, if the balloon inflated during any part of systole.

One additional question often troubles the house officer, namely, the evaluation of the arterial trace during IABP support (Fig. 8.2). On the arterial trace in the patient without the IABP, the pressure spike representing left ventricular systole is followed by a small dicrotic notch (Fig. 8.2, top). In the patient with the IABP functioning, a second major spike follows the left ventricular systolic spike (Fig. 8.2, middle). This

(systole shaded)

FIG. 8.2. Common patterns in arterial pressure trace with the IABP. Top: No IABP. Middle: IABP operating in a patient with poor LV function. Bottom: IABP functioning in a patient with good LV function. Shading marks mechanical systole.

represents inflation of the balloon, with the expected rise in aortic diastolic pressure. This IABP spike is often higher than the left ventricular systolic spike. The automatic pressure monitor that reads the patient's arterial pressure at the bedside reads the highest spike as "systolic" pressure. However, **with the IABP functioning, "systolic" (peak) pressure is transferred to diastole.**

In patients with good or adequate cardiac output, the IABP spike will not always exceed or reach that of left ventricular systole (Fig. 8.2, bottom). This is seen at times in patients who have had the IABP placed for angina rather than for cardiogenic shock. Failure of the IABP spike to exceed that of native systole need not, in and of itself, be cause for concern and may be entirely consistent with good IABP function and excellent augmentation. Note again that this second pressure spike, the IABP spike, represents pressure generated in diastole by the balloon at no expense to the heart. This will raise mean aortic pressure significantly, with consequently improved organ perfusion.

In fact, comparing the IABP spike to the native left ventricular spike has been used to calculate cardiac output. Because the volume of balloon inflation is precisely known, left ventricular stroke volume can be inferred (9,10). Calculation of cardiac output by this method has been shown to be very accurate. A small native spike with a tall IABP spike (Fig. 8.2, middle) implies a native stroke volume considerably below the 40 cc of the IABP—that is, poor left ventricular function.

The IABP is usually used for a few days only, since prolonged use frequently leads to major complications. Limb ischemia, blood element destruction, thrombosis with embolization, and sepsis become increasing concerns. (In rare cases, the IABP has been left in place for a month or more.) In cases of postoperative low cardiac output, recovery is usually complete within 72 h.

IABP support should not be withdrawn abruptly. Rather, the patient is gradually weaned from the IABP. Usually, this is done by reducing the pumping rate from 1:1 (augmentation with every heartbeat) to 1:2 (augmentation with every other heartbeat) to 1:4 (augmentation with every fourth heartbeat). Another approach to weaning reduces the volume of balloon inflation progressively (from 40 to 30 to 20 ml). Cardiac function is assessed carefully at each stage, including determinations of pulmonary capillary wedge pressure, cardiac output, and mixed venous pO_2. Weaning proceeds if cardiac function remains satisfactory. The IABP is removed if function is satisfactory on 1:4 or at inflation to 20 ml.

Experience is required before the house officer will be comfortable with the IABP. Bearing in mind the principles enumerated should allow easier familiarity. Study of the operator's manual for each IABP console type is also essential.

REFERENCES

1. Berger R. Circulatory assistance with intra-aortic balloon counterpulsation. In: Berk J, Sampliner S, Artz J, Vinocur B, eds. *Handbook of critical care.* Boston: Little, Brown; 1976.
2. Bregman D, Hawbert S, Self M. Intra-aortic balloon counterpulsation: a primer. *J Cardiovasc Med* 1984;(August):607–615.
3. Mueller H. Intra-aortic balloon pumping at the community hospital: a matter of qualifications and communications. *Cardiac Assists* 1984;(June):1–6.
4. Reemtsma K, Bregman D, Cohen S. Mechanical circulatory support. In: Shoemaker W, Thompson C, Holbook P, eds. *Textbook of critical care.* Philadelphia: WB Saunders; 1984:482–489.
5. Elefteriades JA, Solomon LW, Salazar A, Batsford WP, Baldwin JC, Kopf GS. Linear LV aneurysmectomy: modern imaging studies reveal improved morphology and function. *Ann Thorac Surg* 1993;56: 242–252.
6. Elefteriades JA, Tollis G, Levi EK, Mills K, Zaret BL. Coronary artery bypass surgery in severe left ventricular dysfunction: excellent survival with improved ejection fraction and functional state. *JACC* 1993;22(5):1411–1417.
7. Beckman CB, Geha AS, Hammond GL, Baue A. Results and complications of intra-aortic balloon counterpulsation. *Ann Thorac Surg* 1977;24:550–559.
8. Lundell DC, Hammond GL, Geha AS, et al. Randomized comparison of the modified wire-guided and standard intra-aortic balloon catheters. *J Thorac Cardiovasc Surg* 1981;81:297–301.
9. Roche Medical Electronics. Intra-aortic balloon pump: model 10, operator's manual.
10. Herzlinger GA. Absolute determination of cardiac output in intra-aortic balloon pumped patients using the radial arterial pressure trace. *Circulation* 1976;53:417–421.

SUGGESTED FURTHER READING

Bolooki H. *Clinical application of intra-aortic balloon pump.* Mount Kisco, NY: Futura; 1984.

A comprehensive and clearly written text, with much important general information on care of critically ill patients.

9 Cardiac Assist Devices

In past years, if a postinfarction or postcardiac surgery patient demonstrated inadequate cardiac pump function despite inotropic and intra-aortic balloon pump support, all was lost. Currently, however, a variety of advanced cardiac assist devices are available that can take over the workload of the circulation temporarily (until improvement is realized or cardiac transplantation is performed) or even permanently (as a permanent left heart replacement) (2). The devices in current use are all designed to replace a single ventricle only. The early U.S. experience with total replacement by an artificial heart (Jarvik) was fraught with difficulties, especially infection and stroke. Accordingly, government and medicine have shifted the focus to univentricular assist devices. The present chapter provides an overview for the house officer of the settings in which application of cardiac assist devices is appropriate and the technological devices are available.

TEMPORARY CARDIAC ASSISTANCE

A massive myocardial infarction can produce cardiogenic shock, especially if more than 40% of the left ventricular muscle is destroyed. Shock is quite common as well after open-heart surgery—so-called *postcardiotomy shock*—and is seen in about one of every 25 cases. This phenomenon may occur unexpectedly, even in patients without underlying left ventricular dysfunction, even when the conduct of the operation has not been troublesome in any way. It is postulated that inadequacy of myocardial protection (cardioplegia), uncorrected ischemia, coronary artery spasm, air or particulate embolization to the coronary arteries, and myocardial edema and/or hemorrhage may be important factors. Experience has shown that dysfunction in such cases is often reversible if cardiac performance can be augmented temporarily. In fact, in most cases where recovery occurs, this recovery is complete, with restoration of normal or near normal left ventricular function. Cardiac performance is most commonly supported temporarily by inotropic medication. (See Chapter 7.) If this is inadequate, then the intra-aortic balloon pump is applied. (See Chapter 8.) This remarkably efficacious device salvages nearly one-half of patients with postcardiotomy shock.

When inotropic medications and the intra-aortic balloon pump do not suffice to restore life-supporting vital signs, cardiac assist devices need to be considered. Without the application of these devices, the outcome is lethal. **The cardiac assist device serves two general purposes: (1) to supply the systemic circulation to vital organs** during the period that myocardial performance is inadequate, **and (2) to unload the left ventricle**, decreasing its oxygen requirements, so that recovery of dysfunctional but viable myocardium is permitted or enhanced.

Similar circumstances necessitating the application of cardiac assist device support may arise not only in the cardiac operating room, but also in the coronary care unit, with refractory postmyocardial infarction shock.

The criteria for application of left ventricular assistance are quite specific: BP < 90 mm Hg systolic and CI (cardiac index) < 1.8 liters/min/m² despite a left atrial pressure of 25 mm Hg on maximal inotropic and intra-aortic balloon pump support. The left atrial pressure criterion indicates inadequate pump function despite maximum volume repletion.

Of course, certain patients are not suitable candidates for such aggressive support measures, including the elderly (over age 70), those with a limited life expectancy (malignancy or other severe illness), those with uncontrollable hemorrhage as the major cause of intraoperative instability, those whose underlying cardiac condition is nonremediable in the long term, and those with irreversible dysfunction of noncardiac organs (especially lungs, brain, liver, and kidneys).

In some patients, not only left, but also right ventricular function is inadequate after cardiopulmonary bypass. Biventricular support with a left and a right ventricular device may be necessary. Criteria for right ventricular assistance parallel those for left ventricular assistance: a cardiac index of less than 1.8 liters/min/m² despite a right atrial pressure of 20 mm Hg.

Several general types of mechanical devices are available for cardiac assistance (see Figs. 9.1–9.4):

1. **Roller-type pumps**. These are essentially the pump heads of the heart-lung machine. They can be used as assist devices to propel blood, usually from the left atrium to the aorta.
2. **Centrifugal pumps**. The "Biomedicus Pump" is the prime example. These pumps are more favorable to the formed elements of the blood in long-term application.
3. **Accessory ventricles**. These "partial artificial hearts" are actually implanted inside the body and driven by pressure lines or electrical connections that pass through the body wall to a console outside the body. The Novacor is one of the most widely used. Inflow for the Novacor is from the left ventricular apex, and outflow goes to the aorta.

LEFT VENTRICULAR BYPASS

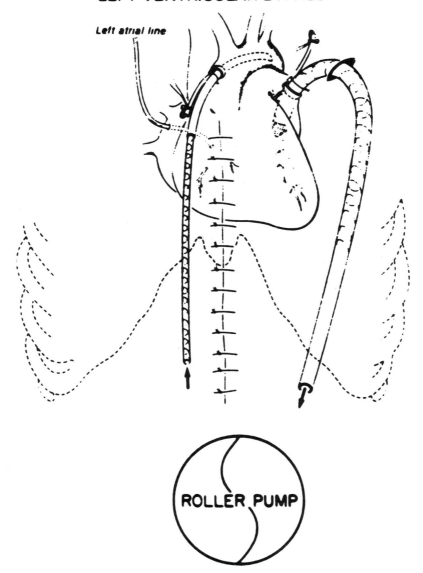

FIG. 9.1. Roller-pump left heart assist (left atrium to aorta). (Reproduced by permission from Ref.3.)

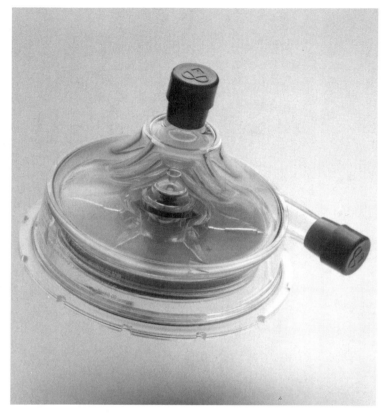

FIG. 9.2. The Biomedicus pump. (Reproduced by permission from Medtronic Inc., Minneapolis, Minnesota.)

4. **The Hemopump**. This is an ingenious new device with great promise. The device incorporates a tiny pump working on the Archimedes screw principle. The device is passed into the heart via the femoral artery and rests across the aortic valve. It can pump up to 3 liters of blood per minute from the left ventricle into the aorta. The Hemopump is remarkable for its simplicity and effectiveness. Despite theoretical concerns regarding the high-speed screw (25,000 rpm), hemolysis has not been prohibitive. Early experience, although limited, has been favorable (4,5).

Certain complications regularly accompany use of ventricular assist devices. Hemolysis and thrombocytopenia from destruction of the formed elements of the blood by the mechanical action are common. Postoperative bleeding is **very** common, especially originating where the cannulas attach to the heart or the aorta. The bleeding tendency reflects the adverse effects on hemostasis of the prolonged period on cardiopulmonary bypass that usually precedes placement of an assist device. Sepsis and

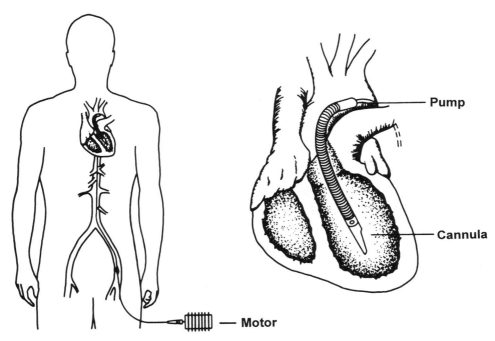

FIG. 9.3. The Hemopump. (Reproduced by permission of Johnson and Johnson Interventional Systems Co., Rancho Cordara, CA.)

multiple organ failure are common, reflecting the very critical status of the patients. The potential for thrombus formation in and systemic embolization from the devices leads most surgical teams to use anticoagulation of some type when the coagulation profiles return to normal postoperativley. This may take the form of Dextran, subcutaneous or intravenous heparin, or coumadin, depending on the patient and the device.

With cardiac assistance in progress, cardiac recovery usually occurs within 3–5 days. The device is gradually weaned and then removed.

About one in two supported patients is successfully weaned from cardiac assistance, and about one-half of those weaned survive to be discharged from the hospital. There is an overall sentiment emerging that **mechanical circulatory assistance is generally instituted too late in postcardiotomy shock**. Late institution carries the penalties of prolonged cardiopulmonary bypass (myocardial and pulmonary edema, multiple organ failure, bleeding diathesis, sepsis). If available, **a cardiac assist device should be placed promptly—within 1 h after completion of the cardiac procedure**—if the patient cannot be weaned from cardiopulmonary bypass by conventional means.

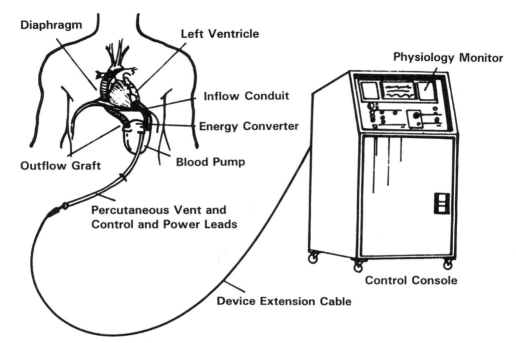

FIG. 9.4. The Novacor (temporary). (Reproduced by permission of Johnson & Johnson Interventional Systems Co., Rancho Cordara, CA.)

PERMANENT CARDIAC ASSISTANCE

In the past, patients supported on a left ventricular assist device who could not be weaned from cardiac assistance died or, if appropriate candidates, were listed for cardiac transplantation. An exciting new option is emerging—permanent mechanical assistance of the left heart.

The Novacor device is soon to begin clinical trials in an iteration that is fully implantable (Fig. 9.5). No lines or tubes cross the skin. Energy is transmitted by an external belt transmitter that is inductively coupled to an implanted belt antenna. The technology to provide permanent cardiac assistance without external connections that violate the integument holds great promise for the future.

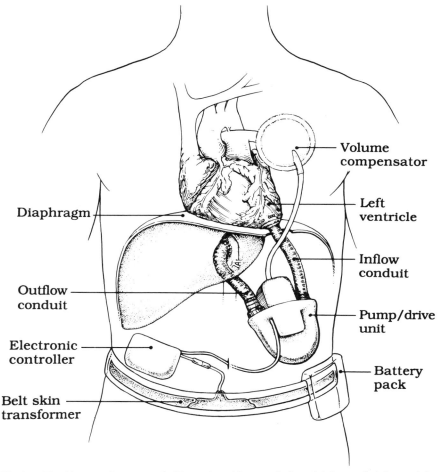

Volume compensator

Left ventricle

Inflow conduit

Pump/drive unit

Battery pack

Diaphragm

Outflow conduit

Electronic controller

Belt skin transformer

FIG. 9.5. The Novacor (permanent). (Reproduced by permission of Johnson & Johnson Interventional Systems Co., Rancho Cordara, CA.)

REFERENCES

1. Bohar RM. *Adult cardiac surgery.* Boston: Blackwell Scientific Publications; 1992.
2. Elefteriades JA. Cardiac assist devices. *Cardiol Clin* 1988;6:449–459.
3. Kesselbrenner M, Bregman D, Sack J. Mechanical Support of the Failing Heart. In: Casthely PA and Bregman D. *Cardiopulmonary bypass: physiology related complications and pharmacology.* Mount Kisco, NY: Futura; 1991.
4. Wampler RK, Frazier OH, Lansing AM, et al. Treatment of cardiogenic shock with the Hemopump left ventricular assist device. *Ann Thorac Surg* 1991;52:506–513.
5. Wielbalck AC, Wouters PF, Waldenberger FR, et al. Left ventricular assist with an axial flow pump (Hemopump): clinical application. *Ann Thorac Surg* 1993;55:1141–1146.

10 Cardiac Arrest and Near Arrest

Much of the pertinent information for management of cardiac arrest is covered elsewhere in this guide. Respiratory management is discussed in Chapter 1. Arrhythmias are covered in Chapter 2. Temporary pacemakers and the defibrillator are covered in Chapters 3 and 4, respectively. Hemodynamic management is discussed in Chapter 6. Inotropes are covered in Chapter 7. Bleeding following cardiac surgery and particular problems that may follow thoracic surgery are discussed in Chapters 15 and 19, respectively. Thus what remains for this chapter is mainly to synthesize material covered elsewhere with particular reference to the setting of cardiac arrest.

A number of excellent guides to the management of cardiac arrest are available (1,2). Newer trends have recently been summarized (3). The present chapter reviews fundamentals in management of cardiac arrest and touches on some controversies and up-to-date trends and recommendations.

NEAR ARREST

The "near arrest" is very common in a postoperative cardiothoracic ICU and not uncommon in a CCU. Blood pressure (BP) may fall for many reasons even in patients who are doing well generally. Intravascular volume may abruptly fall short of the minimum that maintains compensation. Bleeding may occur and lower intravascular volume quickly. A brady- or tachyarrhythmia may develop. Myocardial performance may become sluggish because of acidosis or other factors. Iatrogenic interventions, such as administration of intravenous narcotics or afterload-reducing agents, may abruptly lower vascular tone and cause hypotension. An inadvertent bolus of an afterload-reducing agent may be given as a line is flushed. In any of these settings, the house officer may be called urgently to the bedside because of hypotension. It is not uncommon to be called for BP of 80 mm Hg, 60 mm Hg, or even lower.

The house officer must react instinctively to prevent further deterioration. The general response should be as follows:

1. **Confirm that BP is low.** Many times the arterial line is reading spuriously low. The trace may be obviously dampened; a power flush of the line may remedy the problem.

   With time, the house officer will come to be able to assess BP very accurately by feeling the femoral pulse. One gets to know the "feel" of 80 mm Hg and that of 60 mm Hg. This may save critical time by making cuff BP confirmation unnecessary.

   Quick assessment of the level of consciousness will help. The patient who is wide awake is perfusing the cerebrum adequately, and BP must be acceptable. If the patient has lost consciousness, it is likely that BP has fallen to a critically low level.

2. **Ascertain that cardiac rhythm and rate are adequate.** A glance at the monitor usually suffices. If a profound bradycardia or a serious tachycardia is seen, appropriate remedial measures must be taken immediately.

   Likewise, a rhythm that cannot support vital signs—a rapid ventricular tachycardia or ventricular fibrillation—must be treated immediately.

   Often rhythm and rate will be adequate, with some other factor causing the hypotension.

3. **Take measures to raise BP. Calcium chloride is the inotrope par excellence**. Other inotropes act via their effect on intracellular calcium flux. **Intravenous administration of calcium chloride will stimulate myocardial contractility and raise BP no matter what the cause of hypotension.** Calcium chloride comes as 1 g/10 ml in rapid-inject syringes. One-quarter ampule (2.5 ml) can be given for mild hypotension; one-half ampule (5 ml) can be given for moderate hypotension; and a full ampule can be given for severe hypotension. This drug must be given by central line. Once again, **calcium should be the house officer's instinctive response to hypotension.** If calcium is not effective by itself, epinephrine can be given by injection, as discussed later. Once BP is restored, a thorough assessment can be undertaken to determine the cause of near arrest and to effect a remedy.

MECHANICS OF RESUSCITATION

It is not uncommon to find house officers at an arrest concentrating heavily on the EKG machine and on drug administration yet neglecting artificial respiration and circulation. **Resuscitation is primarily a mechanical intervention: Respiration and circulation must be maintained artificially.**

In the ICU, ventilation is best provided by quick intubation and respiration by bag using supplemental oxygen. (This is in distinction to resuscitation in the community, where mouth-to-mouth resuscitation may be required.) Every house officer must be capable of intubating quickly and reliably. This skill comes only through experience; a rotation on the anesthesia service can concentrate this experience. **One hundred percent O_2 should be administered**. Oxygen toxicity is not a relevant danger in this acute setting. The house officer should be cautioned that in urgent situations it is not uncommon for staff to forget to connect the ventilating bag to the O_2 supply. Vigorous ventilation should be performed. The aim is to provide a minute volume much greater than normal, so that preexisting CO_2 retention and hypoxia can be corrected.

Effective external mechanical cardiac compression is learned through experience. Common errors include trying to perform compression on a soft mattress and being undervigorous. A rigid board must be placed under the chest for compression to be effective. Very vigorous depression of the sternum must be attained; ribs and sternum may be fractured, but this is a small price to pay for sustenance of circulation. **Contemporary evidence favors not only vigorous compression, but also a rapid rate of compression, 120 per minute being optimal** (4).

In the ICU, the arterial line will provide a measure of the effectiveness of external compression. An experienced operator can achieve BPs of 80 mm Hg or more with each compression.

In the patient who is within several days of cardiac surgery, the median sternotomy wound can be opened easily and quickly to provide access for internal massage. It is prudent to splash the chest with betadine before reopening the incision. Internal massage may be done with one hand or bimanually. Internal massage is tiring (the skeletal muscles of the hand are not used to the sustained performance requirements of the heart); the operator may find it necessary to switch back and forth between one and two hands. Again, the arterial line provides an index of effectiveness. The house officer should bear in mind that the heart is delicate. Indiscrete manipulation may produce a tear of the cardiac chambers. Whenever possible, internal massage should be performed by an experienced team member. After achieving successful cardiac resuscitation by open massage, copious irrigation with antibiotic solution should be carried out, and a decision as to primary or delayed closure of the sternotomy incision made; this decision depends on the degree of contamination of the wound.

Without adequate mechanical ventilation and circulation, resuscitation cannot be effective. When adequate ventilation and circulation are provided artificially, the patient's own rhythm, rate, and contractility are, for the moment, not relevant. In this way, critical time is gained to normalize rhythm and contractility, so that the patient's own system may safely and adequately resume circulation.

It has recently been shown that monitoring the end-tidal CO_2 in the endotracheal tube allows on-line assessment of the adequacy of mechanical resuscitation and early recognition of resumption of adequate native hemodynamics. The principle behind this monitoring is that, in the absence of effective circulation, no CO_2 is delivered to the lungs by the bloodstream, and end-tidal CO_2 is low. With effective resuscitation, and especially with resumption of native hemodynamics, increase in end-tidal CO_2 is seen (5).

ARRHYTHMIAS DURING ARREST

The rhythms seen most commonly during arrest are (1) a very slow rhythm (a profound bradycardia or even asystole) and (2) a serious ventricular arrhythmia (rapid ventricular tachycardia or ventricular fibrillation).
The approach for bradycardia is clearly outlined in Chapter 2. Atropine 0.5 mg IV is tried twice. If there is no response, then isoproterenol is given by infusion. If the patient still does not respond, a temporary transvenous pacemaker is placed or external pacing is instituted.

Chapter 2 covers as well the treatment of ventricular tachycardia and ventricular fibrillation. Ventricular tachycardia is treated by cardioversion if vital signs are not maintained. Ventricular fibrillation is always treated by defibrillation. A very fine fibrillation can be coarsened by administration of epinephrine to increase the likelihood of successful defibrillation.

PHARMACOLOGY OF RESUSCITATION

Aside from oxygen, only a handful of drugs are essential for resuscitation (2):

Sodium bicarbonate
Atropine
Lidocaine
Calcium
Epinephrine
Norepinephrine

These drugs are available on "code carts" in prepackaged syringes designed for rapid intravenous bolus administration. Table 10.1 lists the drugs, their prepackaged available forms, commonly used doses, useful actions, and unwanted side effects.

Sodium Bicarbonate

Sodium bicarbonate comes in 50-ml vials with 44 mEq per vial (almost 1 mEq/ml). The dose is 1 ml/kg body weight. This drug is used to correct the metabolic acidosis of cardiac arrest. Acidosis, of course, causes arrhythmias and impairs contractility. We commonly administer 2 ampules of sodium bicarbonate when arrest has been sustained more than a few minutes. Subsequent dosage is guided by arterial blood gas determination.

The house officer should note that acidosis in arrest usually results from a combination of metabolic (from anaerobic metabolism and lactic acid production) and respiratory factors. Vigorous ventilation will correct the respiratory component. It may also be advantageous to overventilate down to a low pCO_2 (25–30 mm Hg) to compensate for metabolic acidosis.

Table 10.1 *Essential drugs in cardiac arrest*

Drug	Available forms	Dose	Use(s)	Disadvantage(s)
Sodium bicarbonate (NaHCO3)	50-ml ampule (44 mEq/ampule)	1 ml/kg	Corrects acidosis	Considerable salt load
Atropine	0.4 - 0.5 mg/ml (vial) or 1mg/10 ml (ampule)	0.4 -0.5 mg; repeat X 1 prn	Corrects bradycardia	
Lidocaine	100 mg/10 (ampule)	1 mg/kg	Corrects ventricular ectopy	Seizures, myocardial depression
Calcium chloride (CaCl₃)	1 g/10 ml (ampule)	2.5 - 10 ml	Augments contractility	Ventricular irritability
Epinephrine	1:10,000 solution (ampule)	2.5 - 10 ml	Augments contractility; restores electrical activity in asystole; enhances defibrillation	Vetricular irritability
Norepinephrine	4 mg/4 ml (ampule)	Give by continuous infusion at 0.02 - 0.2 µg/kg/min	Augments contractility; restores arteriolar tone and increases BP to improve coronary perfusion following restoration of cardiac rhythm	Renal vasoconstriction, increased afterload

The main disadvantage of sodium bicarbonate is that it represents a major sodium load (1 ampule contains about as much sodium as a liter of D5/2NS). Also, overadministration of sodium bicarbonate may lead to alkalosis, with resultant hypokalemia and an unfavorable shift of the oxyhemoglobin dissociation curve. Furthermore, acidosis usually corrects quickly once effective circulation is restored. The recently recommended view on bicarbonate administration from the American Heart Association is that it should not be given routinely (1). Nonetheless, many centers, our own included, continue frequent use of bicarbonate; we do, however, guide therapy by blood gas determination, rather than continuing routine administration at intervals, as was previously practiced.

Atropine

Atropine has been discussed in Chapter 2. It comes as 0.4 or 0.5 mg/ml in vials and as 1 mg/10 ml in prefilled syringes. The dose is 0.4 or 0.5 mg, repeated in several minutes if necessary. As discussed in Chapter 2, atropine is the first-line agent in the treatment of bradycardia.

Parasympatholytic side effects are not of priority in the desperate setting of cardiac arrest.

Lidocaine

As discussed in Chapter 2, lidocaine is the mainstay of the treatment of ventricular ectopy. The dose is 1 mg/kg body weight, followed by a continuous infusion of 1–4 mg/min. In actual practice, we often give 100 mg in a single dose to an adult with a serious ventricular arrhythmia. This drug may be used in the setting of cardiac arrest to help prevent reversion to ventricular fibrillation after successful defibrillation. It may also be used to treat and prevent recurrence of ventricular tachycardia or to treat premature ventricular contractions following cardiac arrest.

Lidocaine will cause seizures in high doses. It can also suppress myocardial contractility.

Calcium Chloride

Calcium chloride is used as described earlier for near arrest. Overuse will result in excessive ventricular irritability.

The appropriateness of calcium administration has recently been questioned (6). There has been ongoing concern about detrimental effects by calcium on injured cells (7). These recent investigations have led to removal of calcium from the American Heart Association's list of drugs recommended for resuscitation (1). Nonetheless, many institutions, our own included, continue judicious use of this powerful inotrope.

Epinephrine

Epinephrine is discussed as a continuous infusion agent in Chapter 7. In cardiac arrest, it can be used as a bolus agent to augment myocardial contractility and to raise BP. It is effective also in restoring rhythm in asystole and in coarsening ventricular fibrillation to enhance defibrillation. On the code cart, epinephrine comes as a 1:10,000 solution. The dose is titrated to effect. From 2.5 to 10 ml can be given. Giving too much epinephrine will cause ventricular irritability and may precipitate ventricular fibrillation.

Norepinephrine

Norepinephrine can be very effective for adjunctive treatment in cardiac arrest. It is usually administered by continuous infusion during resuscitation to restore and maintain blood pressure after an effective heartbeat and ventilation have been established. The patient should be weaned from norepinephrine after optimization of hemodynamic status to avoid its vasoconstrictive effects on other organ systems, particularly the kidneys.

Other Drugs

A number of other drugs may be useful in cardiac arrest. Morphine may be given intravenously in 2-mg increments. This drug is useful, of course, in pulmonary edema. Morphine may help to alleviate the pain of an acute myocardial infarction. Morphine may be necessary as well for sedation in case of successful resuscitation.

Isoproterenol is useful for bradycardias. All the inotropic agents discussed in Chapter 7 may at times be useful.

A number of antiarrhythmics other than lidocaine may on occasion be necessary, especially procainamide (Pronestyl) and bretylium. (See Chapter 2.)

CARDIAC ARREST IN SPECIFIC SETTINGS

Arrest Following Cardiac Surgery

Arrhythmia is a common cause of arrest following cardiac surgery. More often than not, the automatic EKG monitor or the nurse will be able to provide the information that an arrhythmia was the primary event.

Overdistention of the heart by injudicious fluid administration may lead to a vicious cycle of increased wall tension, increased oxygen requirement, decreased cardiac output, and decreased oxygen supply. Arrest may result. Fortunately, invasive hemodynamic monitoring helps to prevent this scenario.

Primary myocardial pump failure may lead to arrest. In some cases, the intra-aortic balloon pump may be needed as part of the resuscitative efforts.

Sudden onset of bleeding with cardiac tamponade is always a possibility in cardiac arrest following open-heart surgery. In fact, in the first few days following surgery, if an arrest is unexplained and ordinary measures are nonproductive, opening the chest for internal massage may be indicated to rule out or relieve tamponade. Beyond several days, bleeding is very unlikely; furthermore, the sternum may not open easily after several days.

Arrest Following Thoracic Surgery

A number of problems may lead to cardiac arrest following noncardiac thoracic surgery. These include postpneumonectomy space problems, intra-thoracic bleeding, tension pneumothorax, cardiac herniation, and lobar torsion. A detailed discussion of these problems is found in Chapter 19.

Extraordinary salvage may be attained by properly administered resuscitative efforts. In our unit, we have had a number of patients survive totally intact following resuscitations as long as 2.5 h. The house officer may not understand the cardiac surgeon's persistence in some cases. It is the surgeon's prior experience that makes clear that survival is possible following apparently desperate circumstances and provides the impetus for vigorous continuation of efforts.

RESUSCITATION BY CARDIOPULMONARY BYPASS

With the refinement of Seldinger over-the-wire techniques for cannulation, it has proved possible to cannulate both the femoral artery and vein percutaneously and use bedside cardiopulmonary bypass for cardiopulmonary resuscitation. Initial clinical success has been reported (8).

If percutaneous institution of cardiopulmonary bypass continues to prove effective, this method may come to represent the ultimate form of resuscitation: Oxygenation and circulation are maintained by the heart-lung machine while the native circulatory system is diagnosed and restored.

REFERENCES

1. American Heart Association Committee on Cardiopulmonary Resuscitation and Emergency Cardiac Care. Standards for cardiopulmonary resuscitation (CPR) and emergency cardiac care (ECC). *JAMA* 1986;2905–2989.
2. McIntyre KM, Lewis AJ. *Textbook of advanced cardiac life support.* Dallas: American Heart Association;1981.
3. Elefteriades JA. Cardiopulmonary resuscitation. In: Baue AE, Geha AS, Hammond GL, Laks H, Naunheim KS. *Glenn's thoracic and cardiovascular surgery* (fifth edition). Norwalk, CT: Appleton and Lange;1991.
4. Maier GW, Newton JR, Wolfe A, et al. The influence of manual chest compression rate on hemodynamic support during cardiac arrest: high-impulse cardiopulmonary resuscitation. *Circulation* 1986;75 (Suppl IV):IV-51–59.
5. Garnett AR, Ornato JP, Gonzales ER, Johnson B. End-tidal carbon dioxide monitoring during cardiopulmonary resuscitation. *JAMA* 1987;257:512–515.
6. Steuven HA, Thompson B, Aprahamian C, Darin JC. Use of calcium in prehospital cardiac arrest. *Ann Emerg Med* 1983;12:136–139.
7. White BC, Winegar CD, Wilson RF, et al. Possible role of calcium blockers in cerebral resuscitation: a review of the literature and synthesis for future studies. *Crit Care Med* 1983;11:202–207.
8. Phillips SJ, Ballentine B, Slonine D, et al. Percutaneous initiation of cardiopulmonary bypass. *Ann Thorac Surg* 1983;36:223–225.

SUGGESTED FURTHER READING

American Heart Association Committee on Cardiopulmonary Resuscitation and Emergency Cardiac Care. Standards for cardiopulmonary resuscitation (CPR) and emergency cardiac care (ECC). *JAMA* 1986;2905–2989.

This is highly recommended for the house officer with interest in and responsibility for ICU care.

Elefteriades JA. Cardiopulmonary resuscitation. In: Baue AE, Geha AS, Hammond GL, Laks H, Naunheim KS, eds. *Glenn's thoracic and cardiovascular surgery,* 5th ed. Norwalk, CT: Appleton & Lange; 1991.

This reviews some recent controversies and up-to-date recommendations.

McIntyre KM, Lewis AJ. *Textbook of advanced cardiac life support.* Dallas: American Heart Association; 1981.

This is highly recommended for the house officer with interest in and responsibility for ICU care.

11 Thoracic Imaging in Acute Disease

Diagnostic imaging of thoracic organs has virtually exploded with powerful techniques in the past decade. The present chapter will provide an overview of available techniques and their application in patients with acute cardiopulmonary disease. Specific references to diagnostic techniques are included as well in the chapters on specific disease entities.

CXR

Having "grown up" in the age of advanced diagnostic imaging techniques, many of today's house officers underestimate the importance and power of the chest x-ray. The chest x-ray remains the gold standard for initial evaluation in the acute-care setting of the lungs (pneumothorax, hemothorax, pleural effusion, infiltrate, mass lesion, cavity, edema), the heart (cardiomegaly, pericardial fullness, congestive heart failure, herniation), the mediastinum (widening, pneumomediastinum), and the aorta (ascending aortic shadow, aortic knob, descending aortic shadow, widening, tortuosity). In addition, the chest x-ray confirms the position of lines, drains, and tubes in the heart, great vessels, and pleural spaces. The cardiologist, the cardiac surgeon, and the pulmonologist rely heavily on the chest x-ray, from which, based on training and experience, they extract a tremendous amount of information.

ECHOCARDIOGRAPHY

Echocardiography offers a wealth of information, is available on an emergency basis, can be performed at the bedside, and is essentially riskfree. Vital information is provided about the pericardial space (effusion, clot, tamponade), about the cardiac chambers (size, volume status, contractility of left and right ventricles, thrombus,

127

FIG. 11.1. Transesophageal ECHO demonstrating flail mitral leaflet (indicated).

masses), about the cardiac valves (stenosis, regurgitation, masses, vegetations), and the aorta (atheroma, dilatation, dissection). With the advent of transesophageal echocardiography, which can also be performed portably at the bedside in critically ill ICU patients, even more complete, high-quality, and precise images can be obtained than with the surface echo (Fig. 11.1). The aorta is especially well visualized. Biplane and omniplane probes are becoming available that improve even more the accuracy and scope of the transesophageal images.

CT SCAN

In the cardiothoracic acute-care setting, computerized axial tomography (CT scan) is most useful for the evaluation of the pleural space (effusion, hemorrhage) and of the aorta (Fig. 11.2). The CT scan, of course, is not a bedside test. Intravenous radiographic contrast, with its attendant risks (hypersensitivity reaction, volume overload from osmotic expansion of the intravascular space, acute tubular necrosis) is usually required.

MRI

Magnetic resonance imaging (MRI) has only in recent years been applied to cardiac and aortic imaging and has proved to be a very powerful technique. The cardiac

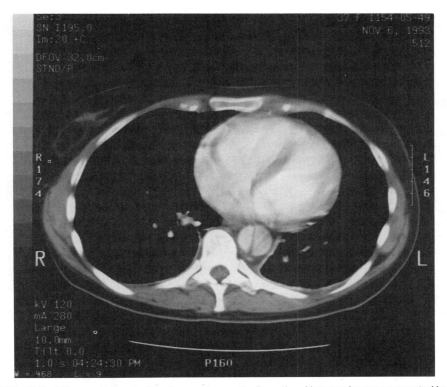

FIG. 11.2. CT scan demonstrating descending aortic dissection. Note two lumens separated by intimal flap.

anatomy is visualized with a detail and clarity rivaled only by direct operative exposure (Fig. 11.3.). Chamber size and wall thickness, especially of the left ventricle, are beautifully displayed. Ventricular function can be assessed. The aorta is precisely displayed throughout its extent. No radiopaque contrast is required. Images can be obtained in multiple planes (coronal, sagittal, axial, and various obliques). Static images are preserved on x-ray-type film or on computer. Exciting three-dimensional reconstructions can be performed. Dynamic images, in which heart function can be observed "in motion" and "beat by beat," can be viewed on video tape or on computer. Preliminary forays are even being made into visualizing coronary anatomy by MRI imaging, raising the possibility of replacing cardiac catheterization in the future. MRI, of course, cannot be performed portably, but requires transport of the patient to the protected MRI suite. Metallic foreign bodies in the chest may contraindicate MRI scanning, because of the danger of displacement by the magnetic field or induction of internal electric currents. Metallic vessel clips used during surgery and sternal wires generally do not interfere with MRI, but pacemaker or defibrillator hardware and bullet fragments do.

FIG. 11.3. MRI image of intracardiac tumor (myxoma in left atrium) (indicated).

NUCLEAR IMAGING

The MUGA (multiple gated acquisition scan) or ERNA (equilibrium radionuclide angiogram) can be performed at the bedside. These nuclear images provide a "gold standard" evaluation of left ventricular ejection fraction (1).

ANGIOGRAPHY

Cardiac catheterization, while extremely invasive, provides essential information on cardiac status. Right atrial, right ventricular, pulmonary artery, pulmonary capillary wedge, left ventricular, and aortic pressures are measured directly. Valve areas are calculated based on pressure gradients. (A useful rule of thumb for the house officer is that the aortic valve area is the cardiac output divided by the square root of the pressure gradient.) The coronary arteries are visualized by selective injection of dye. Ventricular function is assessed by contrast angiography. Regurgitation of the mitral and aortic valves is assessed by left ventricular and aortic injection of dye, respectively.

Cardiac catheterization, of course, is performed remote from the ICU in a laboratory specifically designed for this purpose.

These are the diagnostic imaging techniques available to the house officer to complement his or her assessment of the critically ill cardiopulmonary ICU patient.

SPECIAL NOTE: AORTIC IMAGING IN THE PRESENT ERA

The cardiologist and the cardiac surgeon have long considered angiography the optimal tool for evaluation of the aorta for aneurysm or dissection, especially in the critically ill patient. Aortic imaging is currently in a transition phase in which aortography is to some extent being superseded by powerful modern imaging techniques.

CT scan has been used clinically for well over a decade for aortic imaging. With the use of contrast, the aorta is well demonstrated, but only in the axial plane. In the case of aneurysm, aortic dimension, wall thickness, and thrombus are well visualized. Size estimation is hampered at the level of the aortic arch, where the axial plane of the CT scan cuts the aorta obliquely, exaggerating the dimensions (2). In the case of dissection, CT scan clearly demonstrates the dissection planes—in fact, with considerably greater sensitivity than angiography. In trauma, where evidence of aortic tear is sought, although CT scan can rule out a periaortic hematoma, the technique is not sensitive enough to rule out an intimal tear that has not yet caused a periaortic hematoma. Angiography remains essential at the present time for assessment of injury to the luminal surface of the aorta in trauma.

FIG. 11.4. MRI image of descending aortic dissection (indicated). Note ability of MRI (above that of CT or even angiography) to display entire thoracic aorta on one image.

FIG. 11.5. MRI three-dimensional reconstruction of massive cardiac tumor (teratoma).

MRI provides unparalleled imaging of the thoracic aorta, without radiopaque contrast medium. In aneurysm, dimensions of the aorta are clearly seen, without the axial limitations of CT scanning. In dissection, the true and false lumens and the intervening flap are visualized and their respective flow patterns are demonstrated. In trauma, not enough data are yet available to determine the sensitivity of MRI in ruling out intimal aortic injury.

MRI is becoming our preferred modality for aortic imaging, challenging aortography for this role. MRI offers a clarity of image that rivals angiography. The images of MRI can be taken in any plane preferred by the radiologist or clinician. The whole aorta can be displayed at one time in one image in the sagittal or coronal perspective, in contradistinction to aortography, in which only a short portion of the aorta is opaci-

FIG. 11.6. MRI three-dimensional reconstruction of aneurysmal descending aorta.

fied by a specific bolus of dye. Figures 11.4–11.6 demonstrate the imaging power of the MRI technique.

Transesophageal echocardiography, especially with multiplane probes, provides immediate and sensitive information regarding aortic emergencies at very little risk. Experience with ruling out traumatic aortic injury is growing; a good view of the luminal surface of the aorta at the aortic isthmus is routinely obtained. Transesophageal echo is proving sensitive and specific for aortic dissection. In acute aortic dissection, we commonly perform echocardiography at the bedside in the ICU and move directly to the operating room without any further tests when the diagnosis is confirmed (Fig. 11.7).

FIG. 11.7. Transesophageal ECHO demonstrating ascending aortic dissection. Note two lumens separated by flap.

Multiple recent studies aim to define the relative roles of these powerful tests in aortic imaging for trauma, aneurysm, and dissection (3,4).

REFERENCES

1. Zaret BL, Wackers FJ. Nuclear cardiology [second of two parts]. *N Engl J Med* 1993;329:855–863.
2. Elefteriades JA, Hartleroad J, Gusberg RT, et al. Longterm experience with descending aortic dissection: the *complication-specific* approach. *Ann Thorac Surg* 1992;53:11–21.
3. Nienaber CA, von Kodolitsh Y, Nicolas V, Siglow V, Piapho A, Brockhoff C, Spidmann RP. The diagnosis of thoracic aortic dissection by noninvasive imaging procedures. *N Engl J Med* 1993;328:1–9.
4. Cigarroa JE, Isselbacher EM, De Sanctis RW, Eagle KA. Diagnostic imaging in the evaluation of suspected aortic dissection. Old standards and new directions. *N Engl J Med* 1993;328:35–43.

12 Management of Acute Coronary Ischemia

The acute coronary ischemic syndromes are comprised of unstable angina, non-Q-wave myocardial infarction, and Q-wave myocardial infarction. Each of these syndromes requires acute hospital care; at times the three syndromes cannot be distinguished when the patient first presents. This chapter will describe the etiology and management of each of these cardiologic emergencies. The emphasis is on basic understanding of the ischemic syndromes and on general patterns of care with which the house officer must be familiar in order to initiate appropriate treatment.

UNSTABLE ANGINA

The diagnosis of unstable angina rests upon several clinical features: (1) the transition from a stable exertion-related anginal pattern to a more severe, unpredictable pattern; (2) angina pectoris at rest as well as with exertion; or (3) new-onset angina, which is usually brought on by minimal exertion. The spectrum of patients represented by the preceding criteria is of course quite broad. Many patients have stable angina for years with little or no change in their anginal pattern. Without apparent reason, the stable pattern may become unstable.

Serial coronary angiograms before and after the onset of accelerating angina often show a significant progression in a stenotic lesion. This may represent plaque fissuring or rupture. This finding suggests that plaque rupture can change the geometric shape of the plaque, thereby increasing the degree of stenosis. The development of rest angina suggests the presence of a partially occlusive thrombus at the site of plaque fissure. The presence of a thrombus explains the finding that angina can wax and wane, as the clot may undergo spontaneous thrombolysis. It also explains the progression of unstable angina to myocardial infarction if the clot becomes totally occlusive. In addition to plaque fissuring and thrombosis, vasoconstriction plays a role in the clinical presentation of patients with unstable angina. Quantitative angiography has demonstrated abnormalities in coronary artery tone in patients with unstable angina. Alterations in coronary tone at the site of plaques may initiate thrombosis and in turn lead to more spasm secondary to the release of thromboxane A_2, serotonin, prostanoids, and platelet-derived growth factor. **Whereas patients with stable angina develop symptoms due to an increase in myocardial oxygen demand, patients with unstable angina develop symptoms due to a dynamic decrease in myocardial oxygen delivery.** Symptoms are therefore unpredictable and may occur at rest. The triad of plaque fissuring, thrombosis, and coronary vasospasm interact to make unstable angina a most serious and compelling syndrome.

The chest discomfort associated with unstable angina may be similar to that of patients with stable angina but is often more severe and more prolonged and may come on at rest. At times it will wake patients from their sleep. Rest and the administration of sublingual nitroglycerin will often afford only temporary relief. There is no necessary relationship to exertion. **In unstable angina, the electrocardiogram displays transient changes in the ST segment, with depression occurring more commonly than elevation.** Usually these changes revert to normal after the relief of pain. **Persistence for more than 6 h suggests the development of a non-Q-wave infarction.** The pathophysiology of patients with unstable angina includes changes related to the underlying coronary atherosclerosis, platelet aggregation, thrombosis, coronary spasm, and often plaque rupture (1–4). Appropriate management of this syndrome therefore must be directed toward a multifactorial approach.

Unstable angina is a serious condition, and patients with this diagnosis should be admitted to the hospital. Certain general supportive measures are important (Table 12.1). Removal of the patient from a stressful external environment, reassurance, the display of a competent hospital staff, antianxiety medication, and sedation are all helpful. An intravenous line should be placed and the patient should have continuous electrocardiographic monitoring.

Nitrate therapy is a cornerstone for the treatment of a patient with unstable angina. Sublingual, oral, topical, or intravenous administration is helpful in relieving the vasospastic component of unstable angina and in reducing left ventricular preload and afterload. If sublingual, oral, or transdermal nitroglycerin individually or in concert do not provide pain relief, then intravenous nitroglycerin should be begun. A starting dose is usually 0.5 µg/kg/min, but this dose may be increased sequentially to as much as 5 µg/kg/min. Hypotension is usually the limiting

---

Table 12.1 *Management of unstable angina*

1. Reassurance and rest
2. Nitrates
3. Anticoagulants and antiplatelet drugs (heparin and aspirin)
4. No role for thrombolytic therapy
5. β-blockers
6. Nifedipine, if combined with β-blocker

factor. It is remarkable how much intravenous nitroglycerin may be tolerated by a patient. The dose of 5 µg is equal to a sublingual nitroglycerin tablet (1/150 grain). Therefore patients being administered this dose of intravenous nitroglycerin are taking the equivalent of a sublingual nitroglycerin tablet each minute. (In fact, this may not be quite the case, as nitroglycerin is absorbed by the plastic in containers and in plastic tubing. Also pharmacologic tolerance to intravenous nitroglycerin therapy may start to develop after 24 h.)

Anticoagulants and antiplatelet agents are key components of effective therapy. It has been demonstrated that heparin alone, aspirin alone, and a combination of heparin and aspirin are effective in reducing subsequent in-hospital cardiac events as compared to placebo therapy (5). The most striking effect of these therapies in patients with unstable angina is to reduce the incidence of myocardial infarction. Therefore if the patient is not taking aspirin when first seen in the emergency department, a 5-grain aspirin tablet should be either chewed or swallowed. **Subsequently, the patient should receive 5 grains of aspirin daily. Intravenous heparin should also be started.** A bolus of 100 U/kg will saturate heparin receptors in the liver and elsewhere. This should be followed by a dose ranging from 1,000 U/h to 1,300 U/h, depending on patient size and aimed at keeping the activated partial thromboplastin time (aPTT) at 2.0–2.5 times control.

There has been considerable debate concerning whether there is a role for thrombolytic therapy in patients with unstable angina or non-Q-wave myocardial infarction. The TIMI (Thrombolysis in Myocardial Infarction) III trial addressed this question by randomizing patients with the preceding syndromes into either a tissue-plasmiogen activator (t-PA) or a placebo arm (11). The results showed no difference in the major outcomes (death or myocardial infarction) or in the secondary outcomes (evidence of residual ischemia by Holter or exercise tests). Therefore **the current recommendation for patients with unstable angina or non-Q-wave infarction does not include the use of thrombolytics**. The TIMI III study also investigated whether early cardiac catheterization compared with a course of watchful waiting had greater benefit. The results demonstrated that for the two primary end points—death and myocardial infarction—there was no difference between the two strategies. However, patients subjected to early cardiac catheterization and PTCA, if applicable, did show less evidence of residual ischemia at the 6-week exercise thallium 201 examinations.

β-Blockers have a valuable role in the treatment of patients with unstable angina or non-Q-wave myocardial infarction. This is particularly true if the resting heart rate is 75 or above. Metoprolol (Lopressor) 15 mg IV divided into three equal doses or intravenous propranolol (1 mg boluses) to a total of 10–12 mg will begin to achieve a bradycardic response. Sufficient follow-up therapy should be delivered with the goal of **keeping the resting heart rate between 55 and 65 beats per minute**. The only limitation of the preceding program is the patient with hypotension or congestive heart failure. In the former case, sufficient fluids should be administered to ensure that the patient is not hypovolemic; in the latter instance, diuretics and afterload reduction should be administered to help control the congestive heart failure.

The role of calcium antagonists is more controversial. In a randomized trial of nifedipine alone, metoprolol alone, or a combination of the two in patients with unstable angina, it appeared that nifedipine therapy alone may have been associated with more nonfatal myocardial infarctions within the first 48 h of therapy than in patients treated with metoprolol alone or a combination of metoprolol and nifedipine. It is likely that a key to effective therapy of patients with unstable angina is to slow the heart rate. Nifedipine does not have this action. Studies with verapamil and diltiazem have been less clearcut, as both these agents have negative chronotropic actions. One large trial showed a beneficial effect of diltiazem in patients with non-Q-wave myocardial infarction if there was evidence of preserved ventricular function and no pulmonary congestion (6).

In the preceding discussion patients with unstable angina or non-Q-wave myocardial infarction have been considered together, as it is often impossible to distinguish between them until the creatine kinase-myocardial band (CK-MB) enzymes return. With infarction this test may not turn positive for 6–8 h. Management of the two conditions, however, is not altered, depending upon whether the CK-MB is positive.

ACUTE MYOCARDIAL INFARCTION

The diagnosis of acute myocardial infarction is made by the triad of clinical history, electrocardiographic changes, and serum enzymes.

Despite advances in diagnostic examinations to detect acute myocardial infarction, the history remains a pivotal diagnostic tool. Although a small number of patients with acute myocardial infarction may feel no pain, the vast majority of patients do have clearcut evidence that there is a major calamity. The pain is generally substernal, although it may begin in the epigastrium. It builds to a climax and does not recede. It may radiate to the shoulders, jaw, or arms. The patient is likely to remain still, for even small movement seems to exacerbate the discomfort. Nausea and vomiting occur in half of all patients with acute myocardial infarction. Other symptoms include weakness, dizziness, exhaustion, and at times hiccups. Syncope may at times be the presenting symptom, possibly reflecting ventricular arrhythmias.

The physical examination of the patient undergoing an acute myocardial infarction is important. Patients are uniformly distressed and uncomfortable. They may be restless or remain perfectly still. Patients with acute left ventricular failure will sit up, gasp for breath, and have a dusky hue. There is generally a tachycardia, except in patients who have been taking a β-adrenergic blocker or in those who are having an inferior-wall myocardial infarction, in which case there may be vagally induced bradycardia. There may be a range of blood pressure responses. In general, the blood pressure will be lower than is normal for the patient prior to the onset of myocardial infarction. In some patients, however, because of a profound adrenergic response, systolic hypertension will be present. The carotid pulse will often be small in volume but sharp in its upstroke. The small volume reflects a diminished stroke volume. The jugular venous pulse may be normal, but certain circumstances may lead to abnormalities. In the presence of left ventricular failure, the jugular venous pressure may be elevated with particular accentuation of the a wave due to atrial contraction against a noncompliant right ventricle. In the presence of functional or anatomic tricuspid regurgitation, there may be large v waves. In right ventricular infarction, the jugular venous pressure will be elevated, as it will be in cardiogenic shock. Palpation of the heart may reveal a presystolic impulse coincident with a fourth heart sound. If there is cardiac decompensation, an outward movement of the left ventricle may be palpated in early diastole coincident with a third heart sound. The first heart sound is often muffled because of a decrease in left ventricular contractility. Also, if there is prolongation of the P–R interval, the first heart sound will be soft. The second heart sound may be paradoxically split if there is isolated left ventricular dysfunction. The presence of a third or fourth heart sound denotes left ventricular dysfunction. A murmur of mitral regurgitation may be heard if there is papillary muscle dysfunction. A pericardial friction rub may be present, especially if there is a transmural myocardial infarction. Friction rubs may be evanescent and may require frequent auscultation in order to be heard. A friction rub may be heard on the first day, but more commonly it is heard on day 2 or 3. A friction rub heard for the first time several weeks after myocardial infarction is more likely a feature of the post-myocardial infarction syndrome.

The electrocardiographic changes of myocardial infarction are ischemia, injury, and necrosis; the electrocardiographic representation of these are T-wave changes, ST-segment displacement, and the development of Q waves. Although there is usually little problem in diagnosing an acute transmural anterior- or inferior-wall infarction, there is less certainty when an infarction involves the lateral wall or is subendocardial or nontransmural in location. In the past the development of a Q wave was the criterion for calling a myocardial infarction transmural, and the lack of development of a Q wave denoted a nontransmural or subendocardial infarction. Pathologic studies have demonstrated that patients with transmural myocardial infarction may not develop Q waves and that a patient developing only ST- and T-wave changes may have transmural necrosis pathologically. Nevertheless, in terms of prognosis, the development or lack of development of Q waves does serve a useful purpose. In patients who ultimately are diagnosed as having sustained a myocardial infarction, the initial electrocardiogram is diagnostic in approximately 50% of patients, abnormal but not diagnostic in approximately 35%, and normal in about 15%. Serial tracings increase this sensitivity to about 95%.

The earliest change in a classical electrocardiogram of myocardial infarction is an abnormal T wave. The T wave may be prolonged, increased in magnitude, or inverted. This is followed by ST-segment elevation in leads facing the area of injury and ST-segment depression in reciprocal leads (Fig. 12.1a). A Q wave may be present on the initial electrocardiogram or may develop on subsequent tracings (Figs. 12.1b, 12.2). In patients who have had previous cardiac events, the diagnostic accuracy of the electrocardiogram poses problems. If there has been a previous transmural myocardial infarction, recognition of new injury in the same region is sometimes difficult. The presence of left bundle branch block virtually precludes the diagnosis of

FIG. 12.1. A: EKG of a 48-year-old woman with acute anterior-wall myocardial infarction. **B:** EKG of the same patient 1 day later with evolution of anterior-wall myocardial infarction.

a new anterior-wall infarction. The presence of conduction abnormalities, left ventricular hypertrophy, or electrolyte abnormalities may make recognition of an acute infarction difficult. The diagnosis of a nontransmural myocardial infarction may be even more difficult, for changes in the ST- and T-wave segments are nonspecific. They may occur in a variety of conditions, including stable and unstable angina pectoris, ventricular hypertrophy, pericarditis, early repolarization, electrolyte abnormalities, and treatment with digitalis. In non-Q-wave infarction, the deeper the ST-segment depression and the longer it lasts, the more likely is the diagnosis of myocardial infarction. For all the preceding reasons, the diagnosis of myocardial infarction sometimes rests upon the pattern of serum enzymes.

25mm/s   10mm/mV   100Hz   002A-002A   12SL 108   CID: 1   EID:Unconfirmed EDT: ORDER:

12.2. EKG of a 68-year-old man with acute inferior-wall myocardial infarction.

Irreversibly damaged myocardial cells release a variety of enzymes into the circulation. These enzymes act as a marker of myocardial necrosis and, in concert with the history and electrocardiogram, confirm the diagnosis. They are rarely of immediate value when the patient first presents, because it takes some time for them to reach elevated values in the bloodstream. Serum creatine kinase, particularly the myocardial specific CK-MB isoenzyme, is particularly useful in establishing the diagnosis of myocardial infarction. Serum CK activity exceeds the normal range within 4–8 h following the onset of acute myocardial infarction. The time to peak CK activity varies somewhat, in that—**in patients with neither spontaneous reperfusion nor reperfusion in response to thrombolytic therapy—the peak is at 14–24 h. If there has been reperfusion, CK and CK-MB peak within the first 8–10 h.** The timing of the CK collection is quite important. If the patient delays coming to the hospital, the CK level may have already peaked and returned to normal levels. If there is a delay in obtaining CK levels after the patient arrives at the hospital, the abnormal levels may have already abated. It must be recognized that CK elevations may occur in patients with muscle disease, alcohol intoxication, diabetes mellitus, skeletal muscle trauma, vigorous exercise, convulsions, and intramuscular injections. CK-MB should not be elevated in these circumstances.

For many years, the activity of serum glutamic oxaloacetic acid transaminase (SGOT) was measured. This enzyme is now called aspartate aminotransferase (AST). Levels rise above normal 8–12 h after the onset of chest pain, peak at 18–36 h, and generally fall to normal in 3–4 days. This enzyme has not proved to be of great use, as it is elevated in the face of hepatic or skeletal muscle disease, following intramuscular injections, and with shock. The time course of elevation and fall of AST is between that of CK and LDH.

Lactic dehydrogenase (LDH) exceeds the normal range by 24–48 h after the onset of acute myocardial infarction and reaches a peak 3–6 days after the onset of this infarct. LDH comprises five isoenzymes. The heart contains principally LDH_1, whereas liver and skeletal muscle contain primarily LDH_4 and LDH_5. Elevations of LDH and the ratio of LDH_1 to total LDH are helpful in making the diagnosis of acute myocardial infarction. Abnormalities of CK-MB and total CK in conjunction with abnormalities in LDH_1 and total LDH make the diagnosis of myocardial infarction more secure when the electrocardiogram might be nondiagnostic because of bundle branch block or previous myocardial infarction.

The initial diagnosis of a myocardial infarction must be made based on the history and the presenting electrocardiogram. The physician must then make critical judgments concerning early therapy. Since thrombolytic therapy is most useful when given early and its efficacy diminishes when administration is delayed, correct early diagnosis is essential. Conversely, a number of conditions that may simulate myocardial infarction—such as acute aortic dissection, acute pericarditis, perforated ulcer, or cholecystitis—may be converted into lethal problems by the inappropriate administration of thrombolytics.

Patients with suspected acute myocardial infarction must be admitted to the hospital, preferably to a coronary care unit. An intravenous line is established and continuous electrocardiographic monitoring is begun. Adequate pain relief and sedation are essential. **One of the first measures that can be undertaken in a patient presenting with an acute myocardial infarction is the administration of aspirin.** A 325-mg tablet can be chewed or swallowed. **It is now fully accepted that thrombolytic therapy should be instituted in any patient presenting within 6 h of the onset of acute myocardial infarction who has clearcut ST-segment elevation on the electrocardiogram and has no obvious contraindications.** As indicated previously, there has been no evidence that patients with ST-segment depression should receive thrombolytics.

The recent GUSTO trial compared the efficacy of accelerated t-PA and streptokinase (7,8). The 30-day mortality in patients receiving t-PA was 6.3%, compared to the 30-day mortality of patients receiving streptokinase of 7.3%. In this trial t-PA was administered using the front-loaded regimen of Neuhaus. A bolus dose of 15 mg is administered followed by 0.75 mg/kg of body weight over a 30-min period, not to exceed 50 mg, and 0.5 mg/kg, up to 35 mg, over the next 60 min. Simultaneously, an intravenous dose of heparin in a bolus of 5,000 U was given, followed by an infusion of 1,000 U/h. The dose was adjusted to raise the activated partial-thromboplastin time to between 60 and 85 sec. Streptokinase was administered in a dose of 1.5 million U over a 60-min period with the same intravenous heparin regimen. For patients without a contraindication to α-blockers, 5 mg of intravenous atenolol was given in two divided doses, followed by oral therapy with 50–100 mg daily.

An alternative, equally effective approach to the treatment of acute myocardial infarction is immediate coronary angioplasty (9). The limiting factor in delivering immediate coronary angioplasty is the unavailability of a cardiac catheterization laboratory and/or surgical backup at the time needed. Since thrombolysis has been shown to be equally effective, a delay in its use is not warranted in order to get to the catheterization laboratory. **In situations where coronary angioplasty can be performed rapidly and safely, where there are contraindications to thrombolysis, or where the patient is experiencing cardiogenic shock, immediate angioplasty should be considered.**

If thrombolytics are not administered, patients should be given intravenous heparin in the same dosage as described earlier in this chapter for patients with unstable angina. Intravenous nitrates have been shown to help patients with evolving myocardial infarction. The dose must be titrated in order to prevent reflex tachycardia or arterial hypotension. One recommended regimen is to use an initial infusion rate of 10 μg/min, with stepwise increases of 10 μg/min until the mean arterial blood pressure is reduced by 10% of its baseline level.

Unless there is a contraindication, patients should receive a β-blocker. These agents reduce cardiac output, heart rate, blood pressure, and tension-time index levels. A number of randomized trials have shown benefit with this therapy. In patients with acute myocardial infarction who have not received β-blockers in the preceding 24 h, this therapy can be administered as metoprolol 15 mg intravenously, divided into three equal doses given at 2- to 5-min intervals. While the patient is receiving this initial therapy, evidence of unwanted side effects—such as second- or third-degree AV block, rales, bradycardia less than 50 beats per minute, systolic blood pressure less than 90–95 mm Hg, or rise in pulmonary wedge pressure if a Swan-Ganz catheter is in place—would indicate cessation of this therapy. Alternative β-blockers could be atenolol 5 mg administered in divided doses or propranolol 10–12 mg in divided doses over the course of an hour. Oral therapy with a β-blocker can be continued on the following day.

Although there was once enthusiasm for the routine prophylactic use of lidocaine, this therapy is not now routinely utilized for prophylaxis and is reserved for patients who actually develop ventricular ectopy. A bolus of 75 mg followed by an infusion between 1 and 4 mg/min will generally control ectopy. Lidocaine toxicity must be considered if the higher infusion rates are used for any length of time.

Experience with calcium entry blockers in patients with acute myocardial infarction has been disappointing. Nifedipine used alone, in a trial comparing its effect with that of metoprolol, demonstrated not only a lack of benefit but possibly an increased risk of mortality. Studies of verapamil and diltiazem have suggested that they may reduce mortality in patients without heart failure.

The subjects of hemodynamic monitoring, treatment of arrhythmias, and use of the intra-aortic balloon are covered in other chapters of this book and are not discussed here.

There is considerable debate surrounding whether all patients require cardiac catheterization after myocardial infarction. Although there are cogent reasons proposed by those in favor, the TIMI II trial (10) showed that **in patients who received thrombolysis (t-PA), a strategy of routine cardiac catheterization and PTCA did not offer any benefit regarding death or recurrent myocardial infarction compared with a conservative strategy of performing these procedures only in those patients with recurrent chest pain in the hospital or a positive stress test at a low workload, prior to discharge.**

REFERENCES

1. Davis MJ, Thomas AC. Plaque fissuring: the cause of acute myocardial infarction, sudden ischemic death and crescendo angina. *Br Heart J* 1985;53:363–373.
2. Falk E. Morphologic features of unstable atherothrombotic plaques underlying acute coronary syndromes. *Am J Cardiol* 1989;63:114E–120E.
3. Holmes DR, Jr., Hartzler GO, Smith HC, Fuster V. Coronary artery thrombosis in patients with unstable angina. *Br Heart J* 1981;45:411–416.
4. Lam JYT, Chesebro JH, Steele PM, et al. Is vasospasm related to platelet deposition? Relationship in a porcine preparation of arterial injury in vivo. *Circulation* 1987;75:243–248.
5. Theroux P, Ouimet H, McCans J, et al. Aspirin, heparin, or both to treat unstable angina. *N Engl J Med* 1988;319:1105–1111.
6. Held PH, Yusuf S, Furberg CD. Calcium channel blockers in acute myocardial infarction and unstable angina: an overview. *Br Med J* 1989;2.1187–1192.
7. Neuhaus KL, Feuerer W, Jeep-Tebbe S, et al. Improved thrombolysis with a modified dose regimen of recombinant tissue-type plasminogen activator. *J Am Coll Cardiol* 1989;14:1566–1569.
8. The GUSTO Investigators. An international trial comparing four thrombolytic strategies for acute myocardial infarction. *N Engl J Med* 1993;329:673–682.
9. Grines CL, Browne KF, Marco J, et al. A comparison of immediate angioplasty with thrombolytic therapy for acute myocardial infarction. *N Engl J Med* 1993;328:673–679.
10. The TIMI Study Group. Comparison of invasive and conservative strategies after treatment with intravenous tissue plasminogen activator in acute myocardial infarction: results of the Thrombolysis in Myocardial Infarction (TIMI) phase II trial. *N Engl J Med* 1989;320:618–627.
11. The TIMI Study Group: Early effects of tissue-type plasminogen activator added to conventional therapy on the culprit lesion in patients presenting with ischemic cardiac pain at rest. Results of the thrombolysis in myocardial ischemia (TIMI IIIA) trial. *Circ* 1993;87:38–52.

13 Acute Management of Valvular Heart Disease

John F. Setaro
Section of Cardiovascular Medicine,
Yale University School of Medicine,
New Haven, CT.

To maintain cellular viability throughout the body, cardiac output must be maintained. The integrity of forward cardiac output is safeguarded by the presence of four unidirectional heart valves. Regurgitant, stenotic, or mixed lesions of one or more valves may exist in a subclinical fashion for many years but may lead—via disease progression or superimposition of ischemia, volume overload, or infection—to an emergent presentation. In other cases, a catastrophic mechanical valvular event may precipitate a sudden critical illness in a patient who previously had normal valve structure and function. The present chapter provides background data on physiology and practical information on management to allow the house officer to treat valvular disease in the acutely ill patient accurately and effectively.

BASIC PHYSIOLOGY OF REGURGITANT AND STENOTIC LESIONS

Valvular regurgitation (*incompetence* or *insufficiency* are synonyms found in the medical literature) implies leaking, or retrograde flow of blood due to a diseased valve. To cope with the regurgitation (either aortic or mitral), the left ventricle enlarges in order to maintain adequate forward flow (1); this represents a state of dilation, or **volume overload**.

Valvular stenosis, or obstruction to the forward flow of blood, imposes a **pressure overload** on the cardiac chamber proximal to the affected valve. In mitral stenosis, this overload is exerted on the left atrium and, consequently, on the lungs. In aortic stenosis, the pressure overload is exerted on the left ventricle. To cope with the increased afterload and to reduce wall stress by the law of Laplace, the left ventricle hypertrophies (2).

145

When valvular lesions are acute, no adaptation is available, and swift clinical decompensation may be witnessed. Even in the chronic state, dilation and/or hypertrophy exact a toll of increased myocardial oxygen demand, predisposing to ischemia in addition to heart failure.

In the critical setting where significant cardiopulmonary compromise exists on the basis of a valvular disorder, regulation of circulating volume and manipulation of hemodynamics are essential. **A Swan-Ganz catheter is nearly always necessary in the critically ill patient with acutely presenting valvular heart disease.** Central venous pressure measurements do not suffice, especially in patients with concomitant lung disease and elevated right heart pressures on a pulmonary basis. The Swan-Ganz catheter permits assessment of right atrial, right ventricular, pulmonary artery, and pulmonary capillary wedge pressure (functionally equivalent to left atrial or left ventricular end-diastolic pressure). (See also Chapter 5.) The pulmonary artery catheter also allows the measurement of oxygen saturation in several chambers as well as determination of cardiac output by thermodilution. Pulmonary and systemic vascular resistance can be calculated from the pressures measured and the cardiac output. On the basis of this information, volume status can be optimized and pharmacologic manipulation can be carried out. (See also Chapter 6.)

ENDOCARDITIS, ARRHYTHMIAS, AND THROMBUS FORMATION AND EMBOLIZATION

Before considering each valve lesion individually, certain critical general points regarding endocarditis, arrhythmias, and thrombus formation and embolization will be made.

Whenever a patient presents with a new valvular disorder or an exacerbation of a chronic valvular disorder, the possibility of infectious endocarditis should be entertained. Rheumatic or prosthetic valves are particularly susceptible to infection (Fig. 13.1). Endocarditis may follow the placement of intravascular cannulae, for instance, in patients receiving dialysis, chemotherapy, or parenteral nutrition, or in intravenous drug users. Endocarditis can also complicate dental, gastrointestinal, or genitourinary instrumentation (3). Multiple blood cultures should precede the institution of antibiotic therapy if suspicion for endocarditis is high. Evidence for fungal as well as bacterial involvement must be sought. When endocarditis is suspected clinically in a patient with decompensated valvular heart disease, presumptive antimicrobial treatment should be started prior to confirmation by culture.

Disturbances of heart rhythm, rate, and electrical conduction often accompany acute valvular disease. Such phenomena can represent markers of the severity of the pathologic process and tend to complicate management because of their interference with hemodynamic stability, physiologic atrioventricular transport, and appropriate diastolic filling. Control of ventricular rate in atrial arrhythmias (see Chapter 2) is extremely important in the face of acute valvular decompensation.

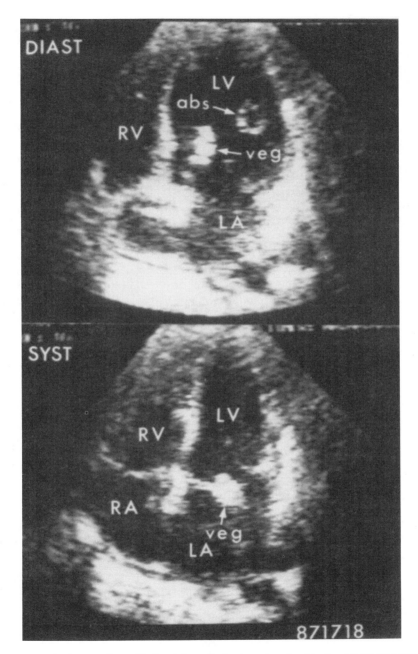

FIG. 13.1. Infectious endocarditis involving mitral valve, visualized by transthoracic echocardiography. Veg = vegetation (on anterior mitral leaflet), abs = abscess (adjacent to papillary muscle), LV = left ventricle, RV = right ventricle, LA = left atrium, RA = right atrium. (With permission, from Ref. 14.)

Abnormal valve structure, combined with arrhythmias and blood pooling proximal to stenotic valves, tends to foster thrombus formation, with possible distant embolization. The classic scenario involves mitral stenosis with atrial fibrillation and left atrial enlargement. Anticoagulation is usually indicated in mitral valvular stenosis, and, in the acute setting, an intravenous heparin infusion to maintain a PTT of 60–90 seconds is desirable.

AORTIC REGURGITATION

Etiology

Acute aortic valvular regurgitation is typically caused, in descending frequency, by infectious endocarditis, aortic dissection, and chest trauma (4). Congenital (bicuspid) or rheumatic abnormalities and the presence of a valvular prosthesis or connective tissue disease can predispose to infection, with consequent valve destruction. Hypertension and Marfan's syndrome are risk factors for aortic dissection, which may extend retrograde to distort aortic valve geometry. (See Chapter 20.)

Blunt or penetrating trauma may cause aortic valvular insufficiency, as can a variety of intracardiac catheterization and invasive therapeutic procedures.

Clinical Presentation

Acute congestive heart failure with a new or intensified blowing diastolic murmur at the left sternal border should raise the suspicion of acute aortic insufficiency.

On cardiac auscultation, a softening of S1 may be heard, ascribable to preclosure of the mitral valve by the regurgitant blood. An apical diastolic murmur (Austin Flint) may be heard, at times leading to confusion with mitral stenosis. The cause of the Austin Flint murmur in aortic insufficiency has not been determined with certainty; it is speculated that apical vibrations from the regurgitant flow or functional mitral inflow abnormalities related to preclosure of the mitral valve may obtain. The lung exam may reflect acute left ventricular failure. The bounding, collapsing ("water-hammer") pulses observed throughout the body in chronic aortic regurgitation are less prominent in acute regurgitation.

Diagnostic Methods

The EKG may show sinus tachycardia and voltage or strain signs of hypertrophy, depending on the chronicity of the aortic regurgitation. Conduction disturbances (heart block) point to aortic ring abscess in cases of endocarditis. The chest film will show pulmonary congestion, though acute cardiomegaly may not yet be manifested. A widened mediastinum or pleural effusion may raise concerns regarding associated aortic dissection. Transthoracic or transesophageal echocardiography will be useful in defining the presence and severity of aortic regurgitation, as well as the presence or absence of valvular vegetation or aortic dissection (Fig. 13.2). (See Chapter 11.) Contrast-enhanced computerized tomography and magnetic resonance imaging are excellent methods for assessing the thoracic aorta, though aortography remains the gold standard for defining aortic insufficiency. Insufficiency is graded angiographically in severity on a scale of 0–4+ according to the rapidity and completeness of opacification of the left ventricle following aortic injection of dye (Fig. 13.3).

Hemodynamic Profile

Pulmonary capillary wedge and left ventricular end-diastolic pressures may be considerably elevated, for instance, at or above the range of 25–30 mm Hg. **Aortic and left ventricular diastolic pressures may nearly equalize,** reflecting the loss of a competent valve to maintain the aortic diastolic pressure (Fig. 13.4).

FIG. 13.2 Transesophageal echocardiographic display of aortic regurgitation by color-flow doppler. **A:** Two-dimensional view of left ventricular outflow tract (LVOT). **B:** Aortic regurgitation (AR) jet. AV = aortic valve, AML = anterior mitral leaflet, IVS = interventricular septum. (With permission, from Rafferty T, et al. *Clin Cardiol* 1993;16:745–752.)

FIG. 13.3. Angiographic view of grading of aortic regurgitation, 1+ to 4+, starting at upper left. Arrows delineate the opacification of the left ventricle. (With permission, from Yang SS, et al. *From cardiac catheterization data to hemodynamic parameters,* 3rd ed. Philadelphia: FA Davis;1988:154.)

Pharmacologic Management

Afterload reduction with a potent vasodilator (such as nitroprusside) is the mainstay of treatment of acute aortic insufficiency. Arterial dilatation lessens impedance to aortic outflow and increases forward flow, thereby lowering left ventricular chamber volume, ventricular wall stress, and myocardial oxygen demand. In cases of aortic dissection, intravenous β-blockers (or calcium antagonists) will be useful to slow the rate of rise of developed left ventricular and aortic pressure. Intravenous diuretics are used as necessary to maintain euvolemia. Oxygen should be administered. **There is no role for intra-aortic balloon counterpulsation in aortic insufficiency**; in fact, the IABP may aggravate left ventricular volume overload by driving blood backward through the incompetent aortic valve. Antibiotics should be started if infectious endocarditis is suspected.

FIG. 13.4. Left ventricular (LV) and aortic (AO) pressures nearly equalize at end-diastole in a case of severe aortic insufficiency. (Reprinted with permission from Ref. 1)

Operative Correction

Acute aortic valvular regurgitation is largely a surgical disorder (4). Refractory heart failure, complications of endocarditis (systemic embolization, uncontrolled sepsis), or presence of ascending aortic dissection mandate urgent operation. Even when urgent intervention is not necessary, early intervention for valve replacement usually becomes necessary because of left ventricular dilation from the acute aortic insufficiency, which is usually very poorly tolerated.

MITRAL REGURGITATION

Etiology

Mitral valvular regurgitation may exist on the basis of rheumatic valvular disease, infectious endocarditis, coronary artery disease with ischemia or infarction, or myxomatous degeneration with prolapse or ruptured chordae tendineae.

Clinical Presentation

The patient with acute mitral regurgitation may present in extremis, with dyspnea and hypotension. The most dramatic presentations are observed with chordal

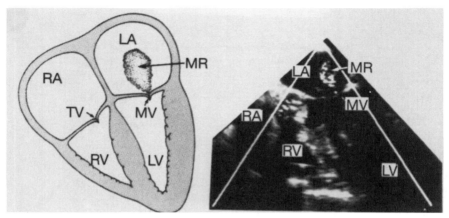

FIG. 13.5. Transesophageal echocardiographic display of mitral regurgitation (MR) by color-flow doppler. LA = left atrium, MV = mitral valve, LV = left ventricle, RA = right atrium, RV = right ventricle, TV = tricuspid valve. (Reprinted with permission from Ref. 15).

rupture, endocarditis, or ischemically mediated papillary muscle dysfunction, necrosis, or rupture.

Sinus tachycardia is often present. A loud, blowing, holosystolic murmur is audible at the apex, radiating into the axilla. Particularly in older patients, the systolic murmur of mitral regurgitation may simulate that of aortic stenosis. A lack of augmentation after a premature ventricular contraction may assist in identifying the murmur as mitral regurgitation rather than as aortic stenosis. A third heart sound and a hyperdynamic precordium may be discovered.

Diagnostic Methods

The EKG is likely to demonstrate an inferior or posterior infarct if papillary muscle necrosis is culpable. Otherwise, sinus tachycardia or atrial arrhythmias may be observed, often with a left axis deviation and left atrial enlargement. Left atrial and left ventricular enlargement, with pulmonary congestion, will be in evidence on chest film. Echocardiography, especially using the transesophageal approach (Fig. 13.5), is an essential tool in assessing the cause and degree of mitral valvular regurgitation (5) (Fig. 13.6). Left ventriculography will provide information relating to ventricular function and angiographic grading of degree of regurgitation, grades 1–4+ (Fig. 13.7). Coronary arteriography is useful in defining anatomic lesions responsible for the ischemic event and guides percutaneous (angioplasty) or surgical coronary revascularization.

Hemodynamic Profile

The ejection of a quantity of the left ventricular stroke volume into the low-pressure left atrial chamber results in a rise of the left-sided filling pressures and

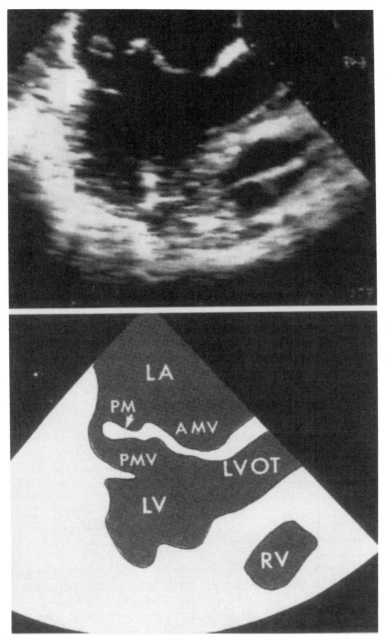

FIG. 13.6. Transesophageal echocardiographic view of ruptured papillary muscles appearing as a free appendage attached to the mitral valve and observed in the left atrium. LA = left atrium, LV = left ventricle, LVOT = left ventricular outflow tract, RV = right ventricle, PM = posterior papillary muscle, PMV = posterior mitral valve leaflet, AMV = anterior mitral valve leaflet. (Reprinted with permission from Ref. 5)

FIG. 13.7. Angiographic view of grading of mitral regurgitation, 1+ to 4+, starting at upper left. Arrows delineate the opacification of the left atrium. (With permission, from Yang SS, et al. *From cardiac catheterization data to hemodynamic parameters,* 3rd ed. Philadelphia: FA Davis; 1988:155.

the appearance of a characteristic v, or "ventricular," wave in the pulmonary capillary wedge tracing recorded by the Swan-Ganz catheter (Figs. 13.8 and 13.9). In acute, severe mitral regurgitation, volume overload may enlarge all chambers until the pericardial limit is reached, causing equalization of chamber pressures in diastole, as would be the case in pericardial constriction (Fig. 13.10).

Pharmacologic Management

Vasodilator therapy, typically with nitroprusside (though in ischemic states nitroglycerin may have a role as well), serves to reduce left ventricular afterload and permits a greater proportion of stroke volume to flow antegrade into the aorta, rather than retrograde across the incompetent mitral valve into the left atrium (see Fig. 13.9). Control of volume through diuresis, although indicated, may be of limited benefit in acute states of pulmonary congestion, and ventilatory support is often needed. Digitalis may be useful for rate control in atrial fibrillation. **Placement of the IABP may be of great benefit in acute mitral regurgitation. The sys-**

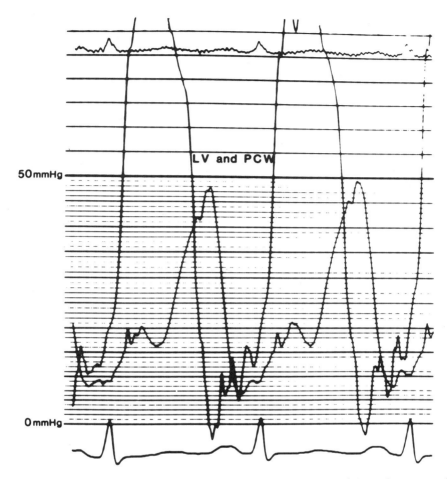

FIG. 13.8. Acute mitral regurgitation with large v wave to 50 mm Hg. PCW = pulmonary capillary wedge, LV = left ventricle. (Reprinted with permission from Ref. 16.)

tolic unloading of the systemic vasculature encourages forward flow from the left ventricle rather than regurgitation into the left atrium.

Operative Correction

Definitive treatment for hemodynamically intolerable acute mitral regurgitation of whatever etiology is surgical, and medical manipulations should be directed toward that end. Current surgical possibilities include valve repair as well as replacement. Percutaneous angioplasty can help to stabilize patients with ischemic mitral regurgitation on a short-term or occasionally even a definitive basis. In any case, surgical consultation is required for optimal management.

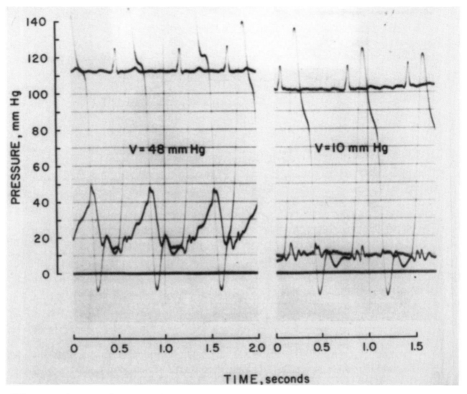

FIG. 13.9. Severe mitral regurgitation with v wave to 45 mm Hg (left) before and after (right) infusion of afterload reducing vasodilator nitroprusside with reduction of v wave to 10 mm Hg. (Reprinted with permission from Ref. 17.)

TRICUSPID REGURGITATION

Etiology

Tricuspid regurgitation may exist on an organic or a functional basis. Organic causes include primary valvular diseases such as rheumatic heart disease, infectious endocarditis, myxomatous degeneration, Ebstein's anomaly, right ventricular infarction, or carcinoid. (When the etiology is rheumatic, there is nearly always concomitant mitral disease.) Functional tricuspid regurgitation occurs on the basis of left heart failure, or primary lung or right ventricular etiologies, which result in right-sided hypertension or volume overload.

Clinical Presentation

Patients may present with markers of right heart failure, including dyspnea, liver enlargement, and edema. If the valve is infected, fever and septic pulmonary

FIG. 13.10. Acute mitral regurgitation with volume overload and equalization of pressures in diastole, simulating pericardial constriction. LV = left ventricle, RV = right ventricle, LA = left atrium. (Reprinted with permission from Ref. 18.)

emboli are observed. If there is a patent foramen ovale or an atrial septal defect, systemic embolism is a risk.

Severe tricuspid regurgitation may present with tachycardia, atrial fibrillation, borderline blood pressure, dyspnea, orthopnea, elevated pulsatile neck veins and liver, and peripheral edema. **A characteristic holosystolic murmur is audible at the lower left sternal border that increases with inspiration.** Stigmata of endocarditis may be visible, and lung findings may point to septic embolism.

Diagnostic Methods

The EKG can be remarkable for signs of right heart strain, atrial arrhythmias, and right atrial enlargement. The chest film shows an enlarged right atrium and right ventricle in organic tricuspid regurgitation, whereas findings of pulmonary congestion or pulmonary hypertension predominate in cases of functional tricuspid regurgitation. Echocardiography reveals right ventricular enlargement and may demonstrate

FIG. 13.11. Transthoracic echocardiographic view of severe tricuspid regurgitation by color doppler. r= right atrium, L = left ventricle. (Reprinted with permission from Ref. 19.)

signs of endocarditis. Doppler techniques can provide an accurate estimate of the severity of tricuspid regurgitation (Fig. 13.11).

Hemodynamic Profile

Hemodynamically, tricuspid regurgitation is notable for an increase in right atrial pressure with prominent v, or, "ventricular," waves in the right atrial trace. Recorded right atrial waveforms may overlap those of the right ventricle to a considerable degree.

Pharmacologic Management

Diuretics to correct volume excess are the key element in treatment of tricuspid insufficiency. Treatment of underlying or coexisting pulmonary disease may be helpful. If functional tricuspid regurgitation has resulted from left heart failure, specific measures, such as diuretics, afterload reducers, or anti-ischemics, should be employed to treat the underlying cardiac disorders. Digitalis may be useful if atrial arrhythmias appear.

Operative Correction

Refractory tricuspid regurgitation, particularly if the valve is the source of uncontrollable septic emboli, may warrant surgical treatment. Valve excision, repair (by annuloplasty), or replacement may be necessary.

(Valve excision, although very helpful in putting an immediate end to septic pulmonary emboli, does, of course, leave wide-open tricuspid insufficiency; this is often very well tolerated. If addicts remain drug-free, they can undergo elective valve replacement at a later date to control peripheral edema symptoms.)

AORTIC STENOSIS

Etiology

Younger and middle-aged patients with severe aortic stenosis have a higher frequency of congenitally abnormal valves (especially bicuspid) in comparison to elderly patients, who are more likely to have senile, degenerative, calcific aortic stenosis (7) (Fig. 13.12). It can be said that the bicuspid valve "wears out" one to two decades before its normally tricuspid counterpart. Aortic stenosis may also occur on a rheumatic basis, in which case there is always concomitant mitral disease.

Clinical Presentation

Angina, syncope, and dyspnea (left ventricular failure) represent the three cardinal symptoms of aortic valvular stenosis. Yet patients may remain symptom-free until late in the course of aortic stenosis. Exercise intolerance and fatigue may herald a major deterioration.

As is well known, prognosis without valve replacement is *poor* once symptoms develop (Fig. 13.13). The prognosis is so poor that most surgeons have had a patient arrest and die the night before elective surgery for valve replacement. The house officer must respond immediately and with fullest attention to any calls regarding the patient with critical aortic stenosis, maintaining a high respect for the severity and precarious nature of the hemodynamic status.

Findings on exam favoring severe or critical aortic valvular stenosis include a harsh, crescendo–decrescendo murmur, heard best at the right upper sternal border, radiating into the carotids, often associated with a single second heart sound. A thrill over the aortic area, a left ventricular lift, and a carotid shudder are findings on palpation, with depressed, late carotid upstrokes. Cardiac gallops may be heard. Typically, the characteristic murmur is easily appreciated. Yet, as with any stenotic murmur, **as the lesion progresses to near complete valve immobility, the murmur may become quite soft—an ominous sign of low forward flow.**

FIG. 13.12 Severe degenerative aortic stenosis, with quantities of calcium in sinuses of Valsalva. Commissures are not fused. (Reprinted with permission from Ref. 11.)

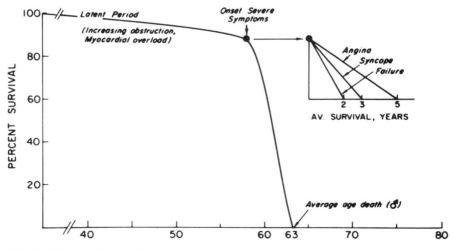

FIG.13.13 Natural history of aortic stenosis. Note dismal outlook once symptoms have developed. (Reproduced with permission from Ref. 20.)

Diagnostic Methods

The EKG typically shows a pattern of left ventricular hypertrophy with strain, and in older patients conduction delays may be seen, ascribable to calcific infiltration spreading from the valve to septal myocardium and the bundle of His. **Atrial fibrillation is an especially unfavorable rhythm in aortic stenosis, given the need to distend and fill the stiff left ventricle in diastole in this preload-sensitive state.** The chest film demonstrates valve calcification and a prominent left ventricle. The ascending aorta may be enlarged, from poststenotic dilatation. Echocardiography is excellent for identifying aortic stenosis and, by Doppler methods, for quantifying the valve gradient and estimating the valve cross-sectional area.

Hemodynamic Profile

Left ventricular filling pressures may be elevated, cardiac output may be depressed, and a major gradient will exist when aortic and left ventricular pressures are compared (Fig. 13.14). In calculations from catheterization laboratory data, valve area is directly proportional to cardiac output and inversely proportional to the valvular gradient. In fact, a useful rule of thumb for the house officer is that the valve area can be approximated by the cardiac output divided by the square root of the gradient. **In an adult, an absolute valve area of less than 0.7 cm² is diagnostic of critical aortic stenosis.** Operation is essential. Valve areas between 0.7 and 1.0 cm² represent significant, but subcritical, aortic stenosis; surgery may be required.

Pharmacologic Management

The patient with severe or critical aortic stenosis is highly preload, or volume, sensitive. The house officer must be careful not to drop filling pressures acutely, such as by nitrate administration. Low filling pressures will be inadequate to distend the stiff, hypertrophied left ventricle in diastole, leading to a depressed stroke volume and low forward output, with consequent systemic hypotension. This situation can create a downward spiral of progressive hemodynamic deterioration that may eventuate in cardiac arrest. Patients with aortic stenosis are nearly impossible to resuscitate, because of the "built-in" impediment to flow out of the left ventricle. On the other hand, volume overload will lead to pulmonary congestion, because of diastolic ventricular stiffness. Thus there exists a very narrow window of optimal filling pressures. In the setting of critical illness, a pulmonary artery catheter will be of major assistance in volume regulation. There is very little that administration of medications can accomplish in aortic stenosis, where the *mechanical* abnormality requires a *mechanical* (surgical) correction. Vasodilators, nitrates, and even the intra-aortic balloon pump have very little role in critical aortic stenosis.

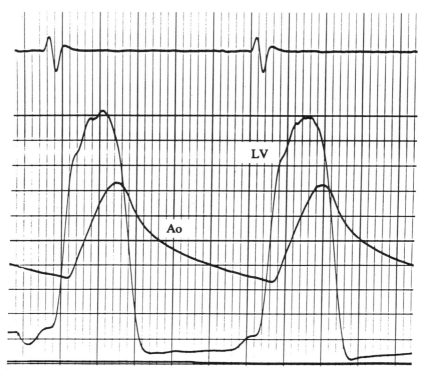

FIG. 13.14. Hemodynamic recordings of severe aortic stenosis, with 60 mm Hg transvalvular gradient. Scale is 0–200 mm Hg. Degenerative calcific aortic stenosis was noted at operation. LV = left ventricle, Ao = aorta.

Operative Correction

Critical aortic stenosis requires prompt surgery. Apart from control of volume and heart rate as temporizing maneuvers, medical therapy has very little to offer. We prefer coronary arteriography, if possible, prior to valve replacement, in order to guide the placement of coronary artery bypass grafts in case of concomitant coronary occlusive disease; not all authorities share this view regarding arteriography (8). Percutaneous aortic valvuloplasty is only of temporary utility, appropriate only for very elderly patients who are not acceptable surgical candidates or who require urgent noncardiac surgery (9–11); results do not last, for no amount of "stretching" of the valve by balloon can undo nature's process of calcific obliteration of the valve lumen. Replacement of the valve with a biological or mechanical prosthesis is essential if the dismal natural history of critical aortic stenosis is to be averted. Life expectancy following surgery is restored.

MITRAL STENOSIS

Etiology

In adults, mitral stenosis most often exists on a rheumatic basis, although over 50% of such patients do not recollect a bout of rheumatic fever. Rheumatic involvement strikes the mitral valve with greatest frequency, the aortic valve with less frequency, and the tricuspid valve with even less frequency. Pulmonic valve involvement is rare.

Clinical Presentation

Typically, patients with severe mitral stenosis present with progressive dyspnea on exertion, eventuating in rest symptoms. Fatigue may be a prominent feature, reflecting limitation of forward cardiac output. Hemoptysis may occur, from resultant pulmonary hypertension. A substantial minority of patients present with pulmonary congestion and right heart failure without clear etiology, and occult mitral stenosis must always be considered in such instances.

The patient with severe mitral stenosis in the critical setting may appear with an irregular pulse and borderline blood pressure with signs of right and left heart failure. A malar flush may be seen, and the left ventricular impulse will not be strong. Many patients will have a loud first heart sound and an opening snap on cardiac examination, and auscultation in the left lateral decubitus position will reveal the presence of a low-pitched diastolic rumble characteristic of mitral stenosis. Cyanosis, hepatomegaly, and edema are ominous portents and correlate well with severely stenosed mitral valves (12).

Diagnostic Methods

The EKG may demonstrate atrial fibrillation or sinus rhythm with left atrial enlargement. Signs of heart strain will develop late. The chest film will be notable for left atrial enlargement ("double density") and pulmonary congestion. Echocardiography, first developed to diagnose mitral stenosis, remains the principal imaging modality for this disorder. Mitral valve leaflets will be seen to be thickened and restricted in their motion. The left atrium will be enlarged. Doppler interrogation can allow an accurate estimation of valve area. In a number of patients, this technique will reveal mixed mitral valvular disease, that is, stenosis and regurgitation.

Hemodynamic Profile

Pulmonary capillary wedge pressure (reflecting left atrial pressure) will be found to be elevated. A gradient will be found between the pulmonary capillary wedge pressure and the left ventricular end-diastolic pressure, representing the

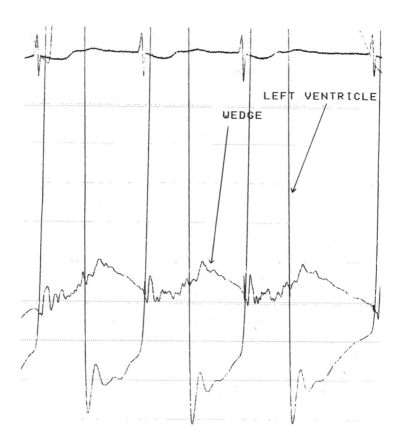

FIG. 13.15. Hemodynamic recording of severe mitral stenosis in an 80-year-old patient with past rheumatic heart disease. Note gradient between pulmonary capillary wedge and left ventricular pressures in diastole. Valve area was 1.0 cm². Scale is 0–40 mm Hg. (Courtesy of Jerome E. Williams, Jr, MD, and Joseph J Brennan, Jr, MD, Yale University School of Medicine.)

restriction of flow across the stenotic mitral valve (Fig. 13.15). Calculated valve area is directly proportional to the measured cardiac output and inversely proportional to the transvalvular gradient. **Severe mitral stenosis exists if the area is less than 1.0 cm².** In chronic cases, elevated left heart filling pressures will lead to pulmonary artery hypertension and right heart overload, although there is an element of reversibility once mechanical treatment of mitral stenosis is carried out (12).

Pharmacologic Management

Mitral valvular stenosis is a disorder of left ventricular filling and therefore requires careful optimization of volume status. **To optimize cardiac output in mitral** stenosis, heart rate, particularly ventricular rate if the patient is in atrial fibril- lation, must be controlled to allow for adequate filling in diastole. Digitalis, β- blockers, or calcium antagonists can be employed. A pharmacologic or electrical attempt to convert the patient to sinus rhythm may be appropriate. Anticoagulation is recommended to prevent systemic thromboembolism. Supplemental oxygen and the judicious use of diuretics are favored if pulmonary congestion is present.

Operative Correction

In patients who do not have significant mitral regurgitation and whose valves are not significantly affected by leaflet rigidity, thickening, calcification, or subvalvular stenosis, percutaneous mitral valvulotomy has proved effective and durable (9,10,13). (In contradistinction to aortic stenosis, the pathology in mitral stenosis *is*, in selected cases, anatomically suited to dilatation by balloon.) In cases not suitable for balloon dilatation, mitral valve replacement is required. This is especially the case for patients with mixed disease, stenosis and regurgitation.

REFERENCES

1. Grossman W. Profiles in valvular heart disease. In: Grossman W, Baim DS, eds. *Cardiac catheter- ization, angiography and intervention,* 4th ed. Philadelphia: Lea & Febiger; 1991:557–581.
2. Setaro JF. Cardiac physiology. In: Bone RC, Dantzker DR, George RB, Matthay RA, Reynolds HY, eds. *Pulmonary and critical care medicine.* St Louis: Mosby Year Book; 1993.
3. Remitz MS, Quagliarello V. Endovascular infections arising from right-sided heart structures. *Car- diol Clin* 1992;10:137–149.
4. Cohn LH, Birjiniuk V. Therapy of acute aortic regurgitation. *Cardiol Clin* 1991;9:339–352.
5. Zotz RJ, Dohmen G, Genth S, Erbel R, Meyer J. Diagnosis of papillary muscle rupture after acute myocardial infarction by transthoracic and transesophageal echocardiography. *Clin Cardiol* 1993;19:665–670.
6. Tcheng JE, Jackman JD, Califf RM, Stack RS. Managing myocardial infarction complicated by mi- tral regurgitation. *Primary Cardiol* 1993;19:40–48.
7. Passik CS, Ackermann DR, Pluth JR, Edwards WD. Temporal changes in the causes of aortic steno- sis: a surgical pathologic study of 646 cases. *Mayo Clin Proc* 1987;62:119–128.
8. Rahimtoola SH. Perspective on valvular heart disease: update II. In Knoebel SB, Dack S, eds. *An era in cardiovascular medicine.* New York: Elsevier; 1991:45–70.
9. Block PC, Palacios IF. Aortic and mitral balloon valvuloplasty: the United States experience. In: Topol EJ, ed. *Textbook of interventional cardiology.* Philadelphia: WB Saunders; 1990:831–848.
10. McKay RG. Balloon valvuloplasty. In: Grossman W, Baim DS, eds. *Cardiac catheterization, an- giography and intervention,* 4th ed. Philadelphia: Lea & Febiger; 1991:511–533.
11. Waller BF, McKay C, Van Tassel JW, Taliercio C, Howard J, Green F. Catheter balloon valvulo- plasty of stenotic aortic valves. Part I. Anatomic basis and mechanisms of balloon dilation. *Clin Car- diol* 1991;14:836–846.
12. Setaro JF, Cleman MC, Remets MS. The right ventricle in disorders causing pulmonary venous hy- pertension. *Cardiol Clin* 1992;10:165–183.
13. Carroll JD, Feldman T. Percutaneous mitral balloon valvotomy and the new demographics of mitral stenosis. *JAMA* 1993;270:1731–1736.
14. Feigenbaum H. *Echocardiography,* 4th edition. Philadelphia: Lea & Febiger;1986:319.
15. Rafferty T, et al. *Clin Cardiol* 1993;16:745–752.
16. Hirshfield JW. In: Pepine CJ. *Diagnostic and therapeutic cardiac catheterization.* Baltimore: Williams & Wilkins;1989:407.
17. Harshaw CW, et al. *Ann Intern Med* 1975;83:312.

18. Bartle SH, Hermann HJ. *Circulation* 1967;36:839.
19. Jaffee CC, Weltin G. *Clin Cardiol* 1991;14:836–846.
20. Ross J, Jr., Braunwald E. Aortic Stenosis. *Circ* 1968;37 (suppl v):614.

SUGGESTED FURTHER READING

Kern MJ, Deligonul U, Gudipati C. Hemodynamic and ECG data. In: Kern MJ, ed. *The cardiac catheterization handbook.* St. Louis: Mosby Year Book;1991:98–201.
Yang SS, Bentivoglio LG, Maranhao V, Goldberg H. Assessment of ventricular inflow and outflow obstruction. In: Yang SS, Bentivoglio LG, Maranhao V, Goldberg H, eds. *From cardiac catheterization data to hemodynamic parameters,* 3rd ed. Philadelphia: FA Davis, 1988;122–151.

14 Arrhythmia Surgery: Postoperative Care

There are two specific surgical approaches for patients with severe ventricular arrhythmias with which the house officer should be familiar: *directed endocardial resection* and *placement of the implantable cardioverter-defibrillator (ICD)*. These procedures are generally applied for patients with malignant presentations (syncope or cardiac arrest) from ventricular tachycardia or ventricular fibrillation. There has been a trend toward use of the simpler procedure of defibrillator placement and away from the more formidable procedure of directed endocardial resection, although a number of centers, our own included, continue to favor directed endocardial resection in selected patients. Directed resection treats the cause—the arrhythmogenic focus—rather than the symptom—the arrhythmia itself. With directed resection, the arrhythmia is eliminated, rather than accepted and treated electrically. Directed resection offers clearcut life-style benefits and possible benefits in longevity (1,2). Patients undergoing either procedure have special needs of which the house officer should be aware.

DIRECTED ENDOCARDIAL RESECTION

Directed endocardial resection is performed in patients with inducible monomorphic ventricular tachycardia, a dangerous but organized and consequently electrically mappable rhythm. Ventricular fibrillation, by virtue of its constant chaotic electrical activity, is not mappable. **The focus of ventricular tachycardia commonly resides in the periphery of a prior myocardial infarction, where the border zone between scar and normal muscle manifests electrical instability**. This border zone is commonly found at the rim of a postinfarction left ventricular aneurysm. Electrical mapping can be done both epicardially and endocardially by sampling the electrogram at many different sites, often with computer analysis of data. The area of

167

earliest activation of the electrogram in ventricular tachycardia locates the arrhythmogenic focus, which is morphologically indistinguishable by any other means (Fig. 14.1). The aneurysm is resected; then the arrhythmogenic focus is excised in a subendocardial plane and lifted away (Fig. 14.2). The ventricle is closed and any indicated coronary grafting is performed.

These directed resections are challenging procedures in patients with left ventricles that often are severely compromised by prior infarction. Postoperative deaths **after directed arrhythmia surgery** are in large part due to two problems: pump failure and arrhythmia. These are the problems for which the house officer needs to be alert. Hemodynamics need to be optimized, by the techniques discussed in other chapters. The intra-aortic pump is often used electively in these patients perioperatively for additional hemodynamic support. The house officer should be aware that observed filling pressures in a higher than normal range (PAD 15–20 mm Hg) may be necessary postoperatively in these patients with compromised ventricles who have undergone these extensive procedures. Also, measured cardiac output often runs chronically at the lower end of the normal range (CI 2.0–2.4 liters/min/m²) in these patients, especially postoperatively. Expectations should be tempered accordingly. Trends in filling pressures and cardiac output are of greater significance than specific recorded values. Interventions should be made to prevent untoward trends in myocardial per-

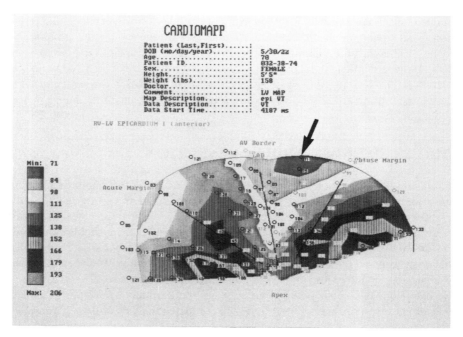

FIG. 14.1. A computer-generated epicardial map of ventricular tachycardia. The site of earliest activation is the arrhythmogenic focus.

FIG. 14.2. Directed endocardial resection. The electrically mapped arrhythmogenic focus is removed by separating the tissues at the subendocardial level. (Reproduced with permission from Ref.7.)

formance. Experienced arrhythmia specialists recognize the important principle that **hemodynamic state and arrhythmia status interact strongly; specifically, impaired or deteriorating hemodynamic status may trigger VT or VF in these patients with underlying arrhythmia propensity.**

THE IMPLANTABLE CARDIOVERTER-DEFIBRILLATOR

The implantable cardioverter-defibrillator consists of a *generator*, which monitors the rhythm, detects VT or VF, and delivers a shock, and *implanted electrodes*, which apply the shock to the heart. The system can be likened to having a doctor and defibrillator "inside" the patient, monitoring every heartbeat and treating an arrhythmia immediately by electrical conversion. The defibrillator may involve *epicardial patches* (Fig. 14.3A) placed by thoracotomy or at time of CABG directly on the heart, or *endocardial electrodes* (Fig. 14.3B) placed transvenously. In patients not requiring open-heart surgery, the trend is toward the less invasive transvenous approach of the endocardial electrodes.

A number of important management principles regarding care of patients with defibrillators deserve emphasis:

FIG. 14.3. A: Implantable cardioverter-defibrillator system utilizing *epicardial* patches as defibrillating electrodes. **B:** Implantable cardioverter-defibrillator system using *endocardial* electrodes for defibrillation (Reproduced by permission of Cardiac Pacemakers, Inc., St. Paul, MN).

- **The defibrillator is often left programmed "off" (inactive) in the early postoperative period**, to avoid inadvertent shocks for the postthoracotomy atrial fibrillation that is so common. (The device counts rate for diagnosis; any tachycardia above the cutoff rate will trigger a discharge.) The house officer must at all times know the on/off status of his/her patient's defibrillator.
- **In case of failure of the implanted defibrillator, standard techniques of cardiopulmonary resuscitation should be applied.** The device will deliver a finite number of shocks (usually three to six) and then stop if fibrillation persists. This is the time for the house officer to take over with external defibrillation and other resuscitative techniques.
- **The defibrillator patches may insulate the heart from external defibrillation.** If one position of the external paddles does not effect conversion, another position should be used. In particular, with right-left internal patch location, anteriorposterior paddle position for the external defibrillator may work best, and vice versa. We use a bedside diagram of patch location while the patient is in ICU, so that internal patch location may be known immediately in case of emergency. This diagram is entered into the patient's chart when he goes to the floor.

Placement of the defibrillator is often combined with CABG, for the underlying coronary artery disease, and not just the arrhythmic symptom, must be corrected in order to achieve optimal outlook (1). Like the directed resection patients, the CABG/ICD patients have most often suffered extensive prior myocardial damage and can be expected to manifest higher than usual filling pressures, lower than usual cardiac output, a strong interaction between hemodynamics and arrhythmia, very little hemodynamic reserve, and susceptibility to hemodynamic and arrhythmic death in the perioperative period. These patients require the house officer's closest attention for a safe recovery.

POTASSIUM, MAGNESIUM, AND ENDOGENOUS CATECHOLAMINES

House officers are acutely aware of the importance of hypokalemia in contributing to ventricular arrhythmias. Hypokalemia must indeed be avoided assiduously in postoperative cardiac surgery patients. In our unit, potassium is aggressively repleted, aiming for serum levels of 4.5 mEq/liter. The polyuria that follows cardiopulmonary bypass may waste large amounts of potassium (often 20, 40, or 60 mEq/liter of urine). In replacement of potassium, in general, the house officer should not exceed 20 mEq given IV over 30 min. Faster administration may cause transient life-threatening hyperkalemia.

The importance of the magnesium ion, especially as regards arrhythmias, is not as widely appreciated. In fact, **hypomagnesemia can cause serious ventricular arrhythmias**. Studies have shown that **hypomagnesemia is ubiquitous in ICU patients, especially in postoperative cardiac surgical patients** (3–5). Magnesium "travels with potassium" and is wasted in the urine of polyuric patients. Magnesium level is checked routinely in our patients immediately after return to the ICU after cardiac surgery. In keeping with published studies, we find levels are almost always below normal. Furthermore, the serum level underestimates the body deficit. We replace aggressively. In fact, in the polyuric patient, we replace even before the serum level returns from the laboratory. We give magnesium sulfate 2 g IV over 1–2 h for supplementation, aiming for levels over 2 mEq/liter. The main serious toxicity of intravenous magnesium administration is impairment of strength of respiratory muscles; this is not usually of concern in the intubated and mechanically ventilated patient emerging from cardiac surgery. All postinfarction and postoperative patients are especially vulnerable to hypomagnesemic potentiation of serious ventricular arrhythmias; this is especially true for the patient recovering specifically from primary arrhythmia surgery. Liberal use of magnesium supplementation is essential. Interestingly, it has even been postulated that magnesium administration exerts a primary antiarrhythmic effect independent of the ion's function in normal physiology (6).

It is well known that circulating catecholamines potentiate ventricular arrhythmias. In postoperative arrhythmia surgery patients with recurrent VT or VF refractory to standard measures, we have had success in our unit with maintaining an anesthetized state to minimize circulating catecholamines. We accomplish this state by continuous infusion of intravenous anesthetic agent (Fentanyl). The infusion is at times continued for 24–72 h, usually with an improvement in the refractory arrhythmia over this interval.

The house officer should take heart that perioperative arrhythmias often do dissipate with the passage of time, usually within several days postoperatively. With the house officer's diligent attention, and especially his/her **prompt, nonhesitating application of defibrillation in case of VF or VT with compromise of vital signs**, these precarious patients can be guided through the ICU recovery and on to safer lives of good quality.

REFERENCES

1. Elefteriades JA, Biblo LA, Batsford WP, et al. Surgical treatment of malignant ventricular tachyarrhythmias. *Ann Thorac Surg* 1990;49:94–100.
2. Geha AS, Elefteriades JA, Hsu J, et al. Strategies in the surgical treatment of malignant ventricular arrhythmias: an eight-year experience. *Ann Surg* 1992;216:309–317.
3. Isleri LT, Freed J, Bures AR. Magnesium deficiency and cardiac disorders. *Am J Med* 1975;58:837–846.
4. Abraham AS, Rosenmann D, Kramer M, et al. Magnesium in the prevention of lethal arrhythmias in acute myocardial infarction. *Arch Intern Med* 1987;147:753–755.
5. Rasmussen HS, Suenson M, McNair P, Nooregard P, Balsev S. Magnesium infusion reduces the incidence of arrhythmias in acute myocardial infarction. A double-blind placebo-controlled study. *Clin Cardiol* 1987;10:351–356.
6. Laban E, Charbon GA. Magnesium and cardiac arrhythmias: nutrient or drug? *J Am Coll Nutr* 1986;5:521–532.
7. Hammon JW. Directed operations for ventricular arrhythmias. *Surgical Rounds* 1986;August:21–29.

SUGGESTED FURTHER READING

Magnesium: the hidden ion. In: Marino PL. *The ICU book.* Philadelphia: Lea & Febiger; 1991.

A clear and succinct account of the homeostasis and physiology of the magnesium ion, including its importance with regards to arrhythmias.

15 Postoperative Bleeding

This chapter looks specifically at postoperative bleeding in the cardiac patient. No attempt is made to review the entire topic of bleeding and coagulation mechanisms, which is covered well in basic surgical texts.

PREVENTION

The key to minimizing postoperative bleeding is care during closure of the chest. Strict attention must be paid to all cannulation sites, suture lines, anastomoses, and vein graft branches. Noncardiac mediastinal and chest wall structures must be thoroughly assessed for hemostasis. The pericardium and the diaphragm are frequent sites of bleeding. The thymus often contains arteries and veins of sufficient caliber to cause troublesome bleeding. The innominate vein and its branches are frequent bleeding sites. The strap muscles at the apex of the incision must be given careful attention. The periosteum of the sternum must be thoroughly cauterized. The bone marrow itself is not often a cause of trouble, because bleeding stops reliably when tight, well-aligned approximation of the bone edges is achieved. Sites where sternal wires pass around or through the bone are notorious for bleeding; these must be assessed meticulously before the bone is approximated.

With a little experience, the senior house officer involved in closing the chest learns to assess rapidly and accurately all these possible bleeding sites while carrying out chest closure. Despite careful attention by expert personnel during closure, however, postoperative bleeding will occur occasionally.

It is known that cardiopulmonary bypass impairs coagulation mechanisms in many ways. These have been investigated extensively (1–3). Major mechanisms elucidated include platelet destruction, impairment of function of surviving platelets, interference at several sites with the clotting cascade factors, disseminated intravascular coagulation, hyperfibrinolysis, and the so-called heparin rebound effect (see later).

175

Bleeding occurs much less frequently than it did years ago, largely for three reasons:

1. Many centers utilize the activated clotting time (ACT) or a similar test to titrate protamine administration at the completion of cardiopulmonary bypass (1). Until recent years, heparin and protamine doses were determined by empirical formulas. The heparin dose was usually 300 U/kg of body weight initially, with 100 U/kg added about every hour during bypass. Protamine was usually administered as 1 mg for every 100 U of total heparin given. Clotting studies, run in the main laboratory, often delayed objective assessment for hours.

   The ACT can be done in the operating suite within minutes. ACT tests during bypass allow omission of routine heparin doses if heparin effect persists. ACT tests postbypass allow precise titration of protamine administration; if the ACT remains prolonged after the initial dose of protamine, an additional dose can be administered. The ACT has been shown to reduce postoperative bleeding significantly.

2. In recent years, it has been realized that many patients will bleed if systolic arterial blood pressure (BP) is not strictly controlled. Also, recent years have brought the realization that cardiac output is well maintained, or even improved, at low normal blood pressures. **For hemostasis, as well as for afterload reduction, we maintain systolic arterial BP at less than 125–130 mm Hg in all postoperative cardiac patients.** It is very common to see dramatic increases in chest tube output during even brief hypertensive crises (as with BPs of 180–200 mm Hg); bleeding returns to normal as BP is controlled.

3. At many centers, a unit of the patient's own blood is routinely harvested via the aortic cannula before going onto cardiopulmonary bypass. This is stored and transfused after coming off bypass. The platelets in this unit of blood will be the patient's own and will not have been traumatized by cardiopulmonary bypass. These platelets can greatly improve hemostasis.

ASSESSMENT

Now, what constitutes abnormal postoperative bleeding? The house officer should realize that significant blood drainage does occur after major cardiac surgery. It is difficult to state numerical guidelines for universal use. Some patients may have almost no drainage in the collection chamber on arrival in the ICU; others may have several hundred milliliters; all may go on to be perfectly dry overnight.

Most patients will have drainage less than 100 ml/h. In general, **drainage after arrival in ICU should not exceed 250 ml/h for more than 4 h** (2). Hourly drainage beyond this limit should be brought to the attention of more senior personnel. **After 4 h, drainage should be considerably less, preferably less than 100 ml/h.**

Even more important than the absolute volume of drainage is the trend over time. The house officer should be very concerned about a patient who drains 150, 200, 250, and 300 ml over successive hours. On the other hand, the patient who drains 250, 250, 200, and 150 ml is unlikely to have difficulty.

A basic principle that must be understood is that **even widely patent, large-bore chest tubes do not drain the mediastinum totally dry**. Some experienced clinicians feel that there is always as much clotted or undrained blood in the chest as there is drained blood outside. This occurs because of puddles, clots, and loculi. For these reasons, the house officer must be acutely aware that **tamponade can occur despite the presence of properly functioning chest tubes.**

If there is any concern about hemodynamic embarrassment from bleeding, the chest x-ray may be used to assess mediastinal size. Although difficult for the beginner, assessment of "degree of fullness" of the mediastinal shadow can be done reliably by the experienced clinician. Here again, trends over time are important. At our center, we obtain a chest x-ray for assessment of the mediastinal shadow (and other structures) immediately postoperatively, 4 h postoperatively, and the following morning, even if chest tube drainage is low.

When bleeding does occur, its origin may be hematologic or surgical. The origin is hematologic if it is caused by inadequacy of circulating clotting factors. The origin is surgical if clotting factors are adequate but a mechanical defect exists, such as an open vein branch, bleeding suture line, oozing sternal wire, or other specific bleeding site.

A coagulation profile including prothrombin time (PT), partial thromboplastin time (PTT), and platelet count will detect most abnormalities of the circulating clotting factors. For routine, uncomplicated, nonprolonged cases, clotting factors are usually normal—especially when the ACT is used to guide heparin and protamine administration. With long pump runs (more than 3 h) and very sick patients, clotting factors may indeed become depleted. With long pump runs, platelet function may be abnormal even if platelet count is preserved.

If the PTT alone is prolonged, this indicates persistent heparin effect. Many surgeons believe in a "heparin rebound" phenomenon, whereby a patient initially well neutralized with protamine may become reheparinized in the early hours after cardiac surgery(3). One factor may be that, as perfusion improves postsurgery, vascular beds that were constricted are rerecruited into the circulation, bringing heparinized blood into circulation. In any case, another ACT may be done to confirm heparin excess. If only the pump team performs the ACT and that team is unavailable after hours, the conventional thrombin time (TT) test can be performed by the laboratory and is reasonably specific for heparin effect. Additional protamine is required for heparin rebound.

If PT and PTT are prolonged, circulating clotting factors are depleted. Protamine alone will not suffice. Clotting factors must be repleted, usually using fresh frozen plasma (FFP). Often 2–4 U of FFP must be administered. The house officer must be aware that the effectiveness of transfused FFP will lapse within hours, requiring readministration, if the body's endogenous production remains deficient. The house officer should also be aware that **FFP is not benign**; it has been associated with noncardiogenic pulmonary edema in postoperative cardiac patients (4) and, of course, presents problems of transmission of infectious agents. **One should not administer FFP to correct clotting studies unless the patient shows excess bleeding.**

TREATMENT

At our center, we often use a paradigm of interventions for the patient with serious bleeding in the early hours after cardiac surgery.

Strict BP Control

In the face of serious bleeding, we control BP even more strictly than usual. We often drop BP to 100 mm Hg systolic by afterload reduction (see Chapter 7). In certain cases, we may even use **controlled hypotension**—dropping systolic BP to 95, 90, or even 85 mm Hg for a brief period. The house officer must consult with a senior physician before using controlled hypotension, as this technique may impair cerebral, myocardial, or renal blood flow. At times, however, 30 or 60 min with mildly low BP may fully and permanently control bleeding.

Raising the Head of the Bed

Venous bleeding may respond dramatically to the simple maneuver of raising the head of the bed to a 30–45° angle. The innominate vein and its branches distend tensely when the patient is supine but often collapse fully as the head is raised. (The house officer should watch for this in the operating room.) Before raising the head of the bed, the house officer must ascertain that this is not contraindicated for some other reason. For example, if the intra-aortic balloon pump is in place, it may not be safe to raise the head, as the catheter tip may be made to impinge on the aortic arch, or the balloon may be made to kink at the groin. Likewise, after truly "open" procedures, many surgeons prefer to keep the patient supine for a number of hours to allow any residual intracardiac air to dissolve; raising the head might allow bubbles to migrate into the cerebral circulation. (Coronary bypass usually does not require opening the heart chambers; aortic and mitral valve surgery and left ventricular aneurysm resection do require opening of cardiac chambers, with resultant introduction of air into the heart.)

Positive End-Expiratory Pressure

Some surgeons believe that positive end-expiratory pressure (PEEP) serves to tamponade mediastinal bleeding by virtue of pressure by the lungs themselves against oozing mediastinal tissues. There is evidence for and against the efficacy of PEEP in this setting (5,6). If the patient is not especially sensitive hemodynamically, we do use PEEP for bleeding patients in our unit. PEEP can be added in increments of 2.5 cm H_2O, from the standard 5.0 cm H_2O used for all patients up to 12.5 cm H_2O. Assessment for hemodynamic embarrassment from PEEP is made with each increment.

We usually do not go beyond 12.5 (or 15 at most) cm H_2O of PEEP for control of bleeding.

Aminocaproic Acid

Some surgeons believe that once excess mediastinal hemorrhage has occurred, with formation of clots in the pericardium, localized accelerated fibrinolysis can take place (5). For this reason, many use the antifibrinolytic agent epsilon aminocaproic acid (Amicar) to control this process. When we use Amicar, we give 5 g IV over 1 h followed by 1 g IV hourly for 5 h (7). Amicar may be harmful in disseminated intravascular coagulopathy, and this disorder should be reasonably ruled out before administration of this agent.

Protamine

In the bleeding patient, we usually give an additional dose of protamine while awaiting clotting studies to look for heparin effect. We usually give 50 mg IV over 10 min. Protamine can drop BP and must be given slowly.

Clotting Factors and Platelets

Clotting factors and platelets are given as required to correct confirmed deficiencies. We occasionally transfuse platelets despite normal counts if the run of cardiopulmonary bypass has been long and we suspect abnormal qualitative function of circulating platelets.

If the paradigm of discrete interventions described above is instituted early when a bleeding tendency becomes apparent, many patients will be rendered dry—permanently so. It is important to realize, however, that no such manipulations will compensate for a major mechanical defect that causes bleeding. If substantial bleeding continues, if the trend is for increasing bleeding, if there is hemodynamic embarrassment, or if a major mechanical defect is suspected, prompt reexploration is indicated. Timely reexploration and evacuation of clots often controls bleeding even when no discrete bleeding site is found. Timely reexploration can avoid hours of chasing bleeding with blood transfusions and clotting factors, which further debilitate the patient. The house officer will come to see that patients who have been reexplored come along well postoperatively, usually just as well as patients who do not have this complication.

Several additional points deserve emphasis. The experienced surgeon can tell quite well which patients will need to be reexplored. One criterion that some surgeons use can be assessed as well by the house officer. The level of blood in the chest tubes should oscillate with each heartbeat but should not advance with each heartbeat. **A fluid level in the chest tubes that advances inexorably with each heartbeat im-**

plies serious bleeding that will not respond to conservative measures and requires prompt reexploration (see Fig. 15.1). Note that advancing fluid level with each respiration is acceptable. We have found this criterion quite useful.

Another basic principle is that **if bleeding has not occurred over the first night following cardiac surgery, it will almost never occur subsequently**. By this time, cannulation sites and suture lines are well sealed by clot and fibrin. In fact, we liberalize our upper BP criterion to 150–160 mm Hg from the first postoperative morning on. By the second postoperative morning, even further liberalization is permissible.

The house officer should be aware as well that, on occasion, especially with turning of the patient, sudden drainage of several hundred milliliters may occur without active bleeding in progress; this may reflect a pool of old blood coming into communication with the chest drainage system. This is seen most frequently when a pleural space has been entered and left in continuity with the mediastinum.

Finally, the house officer should be prepared to handle massive mediastinal hemorrhage when it does occur. Rapid transfusion of blood should be carried out to replace losses. Losses will exceed measured drainage because of sequestration in the mediastinum. Tamponade should be treated with volume and possibly inotropic agents, as outlined in Chapter 16.

FIG. 15.1. The chest tube observation criterion for assessment of postoperative bleeding. A level that rises inexorably with each heartbeat signifies bleeding of surgical significance that is likely to require reexploration.

Massive hemorrhage may need to be handled surgically even in the ICU. **In the postoperative patient, tamponade can be released in most cases by opening the subxyphoid part of the incision and removing the sutures from the linea alba** (Fig. 15.2). This allows free drainage of the pericardium and usually restores vital signs very well. Further surgical intervention can be carried out in the operating room once vital signs have been restored.

When the linea alba is opened, of course, free bleeding to the outside may occur; this may be massive. In an occasional case, opening the linea alba may not suffice to release tamponade. Moreover, in certain cases, massive hemorrhage may have resulted in cardiac arrest, requiring open resuscitation. In all these circumstances, the house officer should be prepared to open the chest fully, even in the ICU, if required.

An ICU caring for cardiac patients should have a thoracotomy set available at all times. In addition, light and suction will be required. The skin is prepped quickly with Betadine solution, the skin and subcutaneous sutures are divided, and the sternal wires

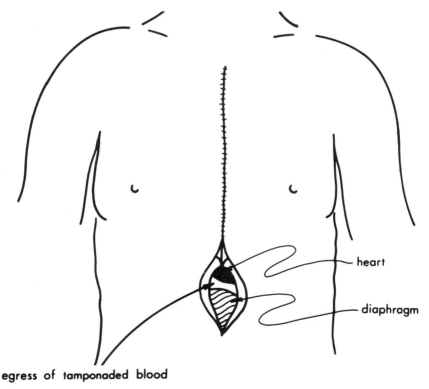

egress of tamponaded blood

FIG. 15.2. Decompression of postoperative cardiac tamponade by opening the lower portion of the sternotomy incision and the linea alba.

are cut quickly with a wire cutter and removed. The chest is spread manually and the retractor is placed. Clots are evacuated manually and blood is suctioned.

Almost all bleeding sites can be controlled by manual pressure. The house officer should avoid the strong temptation to clamp bleeding sites; traumatic clamps can cause irrevocable damage to vascular structures. The fingertip is excellent for controlling aortic bleeding. A sponge packing controls most atrial suture lines. Bleeding grafts can be pinched by finger. When the acute emergency has been controlled, the patient can be transferred to the operating room, where, with proper lighting, suction, equipment, and personnel, definitive repair can be carried out.

Whenever possible, the house officer should await more senior personnel before carrying out the surgical interventions described in the preceding paragraphs. In the rare case when a true emergency exists and a more senior surgeon is unavailable, however, the house officer should not hesitate to intervene as indicated. Such interventions will be life-saving.

Aprotinin

Postoperative bleeding is such a common and troublesome problem that surgeons have long hoped for a panacea—a magic medication or technique that could prevent bleeding problems. An important new medication of which the house officer should be aware has entered the scene—aprotinin. This drug is an inhibitor of the proteolytic enzymes plasmin and kallikrein involved in lysis of clots. Aprotinin is administered intravenously just before cardiopulmonary bypass and then continuously during bypass. (One dosage regimen is 2 million IU initially, followed by 500,000 IU/h.) This drug has been investigated extensively in Europe, with the finding of dramatic reduction in the incidence and amount of bleeding after cardiac operations. The mechanism of this dramatic beneficial effect remains incompletely elucidated; inhibition of the fibrinolytic system and a direct augmentation of platelet function have been postulated. Unfortunately, a tendency toward excess thrombosis with use of aprotinin has been reported, at times involving the bypass grafts and even extracardiac vascular beds (8). These observations have tempered enthusiasm in this country to a certain extent. U.S. clinical trials and additional foreign trials are under way (9). Topical application has been attempted, in the hope of avoiding untoward systemic effects (10).

Although aprotinin may not prove the panacea for which surgeons have hoped, there is every possibility that this drug may prove to be a powerful weapon in the armamentarium for prevention of postoperative bleeding. Even if general use does not prove appropriate, it appears that use in specific scenarios where bleeding is likely to be troublesome (e.g., in redo coronary or valve operations or in complex aortic reconstructions) will be indicated. So impressed are our European colleagues that many would not undertake such procedures without the use of aprotinin. The FDA, based on recent U.S. trials, has just announced its decision to provide approval for use of aprotinin in cardiac surgery. The drug should become generally available soon.

REFERENCES

1. Verska J. Control of heparinization by activated clotting time during bypass with improved postoperative hemostasis. *Ann Thorac Surg* 1977;24:170–173.
2. Cordell A. *Hematologic complications of intrathoracic surgery.* Boston: Little, Brown; 1979:27–34.
3. Gollub S. Heparin rebound in open heart surgery. *Surg Gynecol Obstet* 1967;124:337–346.
4. Hashim SW, Kay HR, Hammond GL, et al. Noncardiogenic pulmonary edema following cardiopulmonary bypass: an anaphylactic reaction to frozen plasma. *Am J Surg* 1983;145:508–513.
5. Ilabaca P, Ochsner J, Mills N. Positive end-expiratory pressure in the management of the patient with a postoperative bleeding heart. *Ann Thorac Surg* 1980;30:281–284.
6. Murphy D, Finlayson D, Craver J, et al. Effect of positive end-expiratory pressure on excessive mediastinal bleeding after cardiac operations: A controlled study. *J Thorac Cardiovasc Surg* 1983;85:864–869.
7. Package insert. Amicar. Lederle Laboratories; Pearl River, NY.
8. Cosgrove DM, Huric B, Lytle BW, et al. Aprotinin therapy for reoperative myocardial revascularization: a placebo-controlled study. *Ann Thorac Surg* 1992;54:1031–1036.
9. Boldt J, Knothe C, Sickman B, Fill S, Dapper F, Hempelmann G. Platelet function in cardiac surgery: influence of temperature and aprotinin. *Ann Thorac Surg* 1993;55:652–658.
10. Tatar H, Cicek S, Demirdilic U, Ozal E, Suer H, Ozturk O, Isiklar H. Topical use of aprotinin in open heart operations. *Ann Thorac Surg* 1993;55:659–661.

SUGGESTED FURTHER READING

Cordell, A. Hematologic complications of extracorporeal circulation. In: A. Cordell A, Ellison R, eds. *Complications of intrathoracic surgery.* Boston: Little, Brown; 1979:27–34.

A concise presentation of the effects of cardiopulmonary bypass, with both a review of the literature and a presentation of the author's own viewpoints.

16 Chest Trauma

The general physiologic management of abdominal and extremity injuries is usually straightforward. The acute critical derangement is hypovolemia. Later, sepsis may supervene. Cardiac and thoracic injuries, however, do not present such a clear physiologic picture. This chapter will clarify the physiologic abnormalities in chest injuries and their management. The emphasis will be on acute management by the nonspecialist that is required to preserve the patient's life until the specialist can intervene. We will not go into the details of operative management of specific thoracic and cardiac injuries. Many of the conditions discussed can arise directly in the ICU setting without trauma per se, and the same principles of assessment and management apply.

Rutherford (1) has listed six general categories of physiologic abnormality following chest trauma that are acutely life-threatening:

Airway obstruction
Flail chest
Sucking chest wound
Massive hemothorax
Tension pneumothorax
Cardiac tamponade.

These are the conditions that can take the patient's life within the first few minutes after arrival in the emergency room. Note that these are categories of physiologic abnormality, not specific injuries. Each category may follow any of a number of specific injuries, and a given injury may bring about several of these abnormalities. For example, massive hemothorax may be the result of an aortic transection from a motor vehicle accident, a gunshot wound of the lung parenchyma, or a knife wound of an intercostal vessel. Likewise, cardiac tamponade may result from an atrial knife wound, a blunt ventricular rupture, a coronary artery laceration, or other specific injury.

The discussion of these six entities will be organized as follows. First, we will define each condition. Next, we will discuss the physiology of how each condition hurts the patient. Then we will discuss how to diagnose each condition within minutes—based solely on vital signs, brief physical examination, and one single radiographic procedure. Finally, we will cover how to manage each condition within minutes.

The one diagnostic procedure required is the chest x-ray (CXR). Hematocrit, blood gases, electrocardiogram, and other studies may prove useful, but the chest x-ray is indispensable in every case.

DEFINITIONS

Airway Obstruction

Airway obstruction is self-explanatory. Injuries to the chest can disrupt the airway in its course through the upper mediastinum. The lumen may be obstructed or the trachea or bronchi may be transected, with loss of continuity. These can be devastating injuries (Fig. 16.1A).

Flail Chest

Flail chest is a disruption of the continuity of the rigid thoracic cage, with paradoxical movement of the disrupted segment. Since the thoracic cage in the transverse plane is a rigid oval, with ribs attached posteriorly at the spine and anteriorly at the sternum, flailing requires that at least one rib be broken in at least two places (Fig. 16.1B). If one rib were broken in one place only, it would still be attached anteriorly and posteriorly. Usually, a number of adjacent ribs are broken in multiple spots, so that a segment of chest wall is free to be sucked in during inspiration and pushed out during expiration, while the intact chest cage moves in the opposite direction during each phase.

Sucking Chest Wound

A sucking chest wound results from a loss of integrity of the chest wall, so that air is free to move in and out of the pleural space to the atmosphere (Fig. 16.1C). A chest tube (before it is hooked to the suction device) represents a sucking chest wound. The to-and-fro rush of air with breathing is one sign that the surgeon looks for to confirm that the tube is well situated in the pleural space.

Massive Hemothorax

Hemothorax is the presence of blood in the pleural space; massive hemothorax is the presence of large amounts of blood in the pleural space (Fig. 16.1D). Massive he-

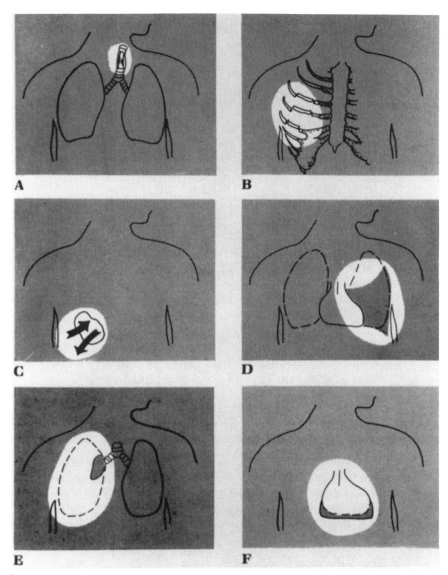

FIG.16.1. Schematic representation of the six major physiologic categories of injury that can take the patient's life within the first few minutes of chest trauma. **A:** Airway obstruction. **B:** Flail chest. **C:** Sucking chest wound. **D:** Massive hemothorax. **E:** Tension pneumothorax. **F:** Cardiac tamponade.

mothorax is differentiated from simple hemothorax because a small hemothorax is not acutely life-threatening.

Tension Pneumothorax

Pneumothorax is the presence of air in the pleural space; tension pneumothorax is the presence of air under pressure. An ordinary pneumothorax is not acutely life-threatening, whereas tension pneumothorax may be (Fig. 16.1E).

Cardiac Tamponade

Cardiac tamponade refers to impairment of cardiac function by fluid under pressure in the pericardial space. In the context of trauma, the offending fluid is blood. In nontraumatic conditions, transudates, exudates, purulent fluids, and chyle can cause tamponade (Fig. 16.1F).

PHYSIOLOGY OF CARDIORESPIRATORY EMBARRASSMENT

Much experimental work has gone into elucidating the physiology of chest injuries (1–4). Both historical and modern theories have been summarized by Rutherford (1). The explanations presented here are purposely oversimplified. By conceiving the injuries as described, however, the house officer will be led to appropriate therapeutic interventions.

Airway Obstruction

Airway obstruction injures the patient via hypoventilation and elevation of pCO_2. Obstruction of the airway impairs movement of air to and fro in the tracheobronchial tree; that is, it impairs minute volume. As is discussed in Chapter 1, CO_2 rises as minute volume falls; O_2 is often preserved until minute volume falls very low. The patient with traumatic airway obstruction will be hypoventilated; in late stages, he or she may be hypo-oxygenated as well.

Sucking Chest Wound

Many mechanisms have been proposed to explain the distress seen with sucking chest wounds; none is totally satisfactory (1). It is safe to say that distress can occur even without development of tension pneumothorax, that simple loss of function of the ipsilateral lung is not the critical defect, and that **some disturbance of the thoracic bellows appears likely**. Tidal volume is wasted moving air in and out of the pleural space, which, unlike the alveolus, is not a respiratory exchange membrane. The bigger the defect, the greater the ventilatory burden. Even a young, robust patient can succumb if the defect is large. **The patient who succumbs to a sucking chest wound dies hypoventilated, with a high pCO_2.**

Flail Chest

The physiology of flail chest is similarly complex. Here, although the pleural space is not open, tidal volume is wasted in moving the chest wall in and out. This movement of the chest wall represents a wasted tidal volume equal to the area in square centimeters of the defect multiplied by the length of its to-and-fro travel (similar to the volume of displacement in a cylinder in an automobile engine, equal to bore times stroke). This volume is lost from each breath, and **in flail chest, as in sucking chest wound, the patient is overwhelmed by the work of breathing and dies hypoventilated.**

Massive Hemothorax

The physiology of massive hemothorax can be confusing; many house officers believe that the patient succumbs because the blood impinges on the lung, impairing its respiratory function. This is not the mechanism. A young, otherwise healthy patient will usually not be symptomatic if one entire pleural space is filled with fluid. Such a patient manages to ventilate adequately with the opposite lung. Pneumonectomy can be done even in elderly patients with poor lung function, and they are not rendered dyspneic at rest. (This situation is not entirely analogous, for in pneumonectomy the pulmonary artery is interrupted as well, preventing the shunting of blood through a collapsed lung.) In any case, **the patient with a massive hemothorax dies by exsanguination into the pleural space, not by restriction of pulmonary function. Nearly an entire blood volume can be lost into one hemithorax.**

Tension Pneumothorax

Tension pneumothorax does not kill the patient by eliminating function of the affected lung. Again, the patient could survive well with just the opposite lung functioning. Rather, **the patient with tension pneumothorax dies from circulatory embarrassment**. The superior vena cava (SVC) is relatively fixed to the adjacent organs. The inferior vena cava (IVC) is fixed to the liver. When pressure develops in one chest, the heart is displaced toward the opposite side. If displacement is great enough, it is thought, the venous return through the SVC and IVC can be impaired. Stroke volume and cardiac output suffer because of inadequate blood return to the heart. Shock may supervene.

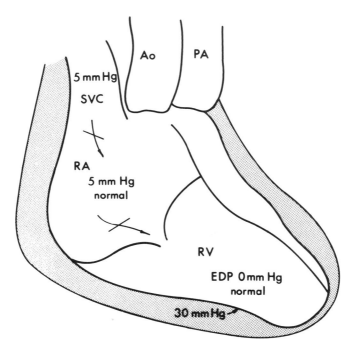

FIG.16.2. Pathophysiology of cardiac tamponade. Normal right heart filling pressures are shown. Blood in the pericardium creates an abnormally positive pressure in the pericardial space. This pressure is transmitted to the ventricular cavity. All gradients for filling of the ventricular cavity are lost. The heart cannot pump because the heart cannot fill. (Consideration, for purposes of clarity, is limited to the right heart.)

Cardiac Tamponade

The house officer may have difficulty conceptualizing the physiology of cardiac tamponade. The pericardial space is relatively inelastic. It is unwilling to stretch beyond a finite volume. As this volume is exceeded, pressure builds in the pericardial space. This pressure is transmitted to the myocardium and to the ventricular chambers. Under normal circumstances, the right ventricle (RV) fills because the right atrial (RA) pressure, usually about 5 cm H_2O in a normal heart, exceeds the RV diastolic pressure, usually near zero in a normal heart. It is this RA-to-RV gradient that fills the ventricle. The RA is in turn filled because of SVC-to-RA and IVC-to-RA gradients. In tamponade, if, say, a pressure of 30 cm H_2O develops in the pericardial space and is transmitted to the RV, blood from the lower-pressure RA will not enter or fill the RV (Fig. 16.2). Thus **in cardiac tamponade, the heart cannot pump because the heart cannot fill**. The patient dies hypotensive in cardiogenic shock.

It will be seen that these physiologic concepts have important therapeutic correlates. These will become clear in the discussion of how to treat these disorders. These explanations, although to some extent oversimplified, have been chosen because they lead to appropriate conclusions regarding acute treatment of these life-threatening injuries.

DIAGNOSIS

Because the traumatic conditions described are acutely life-threatening, their diagnosis must be made rapidly. This discussion will focus on how to diagnose these conditions within minutes, based on vital signs, physical examination, and CXR only. No more sophisticated or time-consuming laboratory tests will be used.

Airway Obstruction

Airway obstruction is an obvious clinical diagnosis. The patient tries to move air but cannot. The respiratory muscles act, but the chest does not expand. Good air movement cannot be felt or heard at the nose and the mouth. One of the major benefits of a rotation on an anesthesia service is that it teaches the house officer to recognize airway obstruction: a stage of obstruction is part of every general anesthetic induction.

Flail Chest

Flail chest is a diagnosis of inspection. Many times, flails are missed because concerted inspection of chest wall motion is omitted. It is important that severely traumatized patients have all clothing removed. With attention to the chest, a flail will be apparent as a segment of chest wall that moves in with inspiration and out with expiration—out of synchrony with the remainder of the chest. This paradoxical movement can be appreciated also on palpation, and rib fractures and tenderness can also be found. Flail chest is not a sophisticated diagnosis; rather, with good observation, it is an obvious one.

Sucking Chest Wound

Sucking chest wound is a diagnosis made by listening—not through a stethoscope, but with one's ear. Once heard, the sound of air rushing in and out of the pleural space with each breath is unmistakable. It is the same sound that is made through a chest tube before the tube is connected. Again, this is not a sophisticated diagnosis. Usually, it is obvious from listening that a patient has a sucking chest wound the moment he or she is brought into the trauma room. From that point on, it is just a matter of removing the patient's clothing to identify the site of the chest wall defect.

Massive Hemothorax and Tension Pneumothorax

Massive hemothorax and tension pneumothorax share one physical finding and are disparate in another. The physical finding they share is decreased breath sounds. The physical finding in which they are disparate is resonance to percussion: Hemothorax is dull, and pneumothorax is hyperresonant. The dullness of hemothorax may not be easy to appreciate in a noisy, hectic trauma room. The severely injured patient will be supine; the dullness of the hemothorax will be, accordingly, posterior only.

The diagnosis of massive hemothorax or tension pneumothorax will be confirmed by CXR, which is available within minutes in emergency wards. Tension pneumothorax is obvious by CXR (Fig. 16.3). In addition to collapse of the lung, one sees displacement of the mediastinum, overexpansion of the ipsilateral intercostal spaces, and depression of the ipsilateral diaphragm. Hemothorax, even massive hemothorax, may be a subtle CXR diagnosis (Fig. 16.4). Most house officers are accustomed to interpreting upright CXRs. On an upright CXR, a pleural effusion shows its characteristic meniscus-type layering shadow on posteroanterior and lateral views. On upright studies, a massive hemothorax would appear just like a large pleural effusion. In the severely traumatized patient, however, the CXR will likely need to be obtained supine.

FIG.16.3. CXR in tension pneumothorax.

A

B

FIG.16.4. CXR in hemothorax. **A**: Upright. Note meniscus of fluid in right hemithorax. **B**. Supine. Note diffuse increase in density representing fluid in left hemithorax.

On a supine CXR, a massive hemothorax will show only as a diffuse increase
in density of the affected hemithorax. A liter of fluid may be just detectable to the
astute observer. Two liters of fluid may be subtle. It is important to be alert that in the
traumatized patient a homogeneous increase in density of one side of the chest probably represents major hemothorax. If the patient stabilizes before treatment is required,
upright and lateral CXRs may clarify the diagnosis.

Cardiac Tamponade

Cardiac tamponade may be a more subtle diagnosis. The house officer should
be aware of the classic triad (Beck's triad) of findings in tamponade: decreased
pulse pressure, distant heart sounds, and jugular venous distention. Pulse pressure refers to the difference between systolic and diastolic pressures. In tamponade,
the blood pressure may vary from mildly to severely decreased. In particular, the pulse
pressure suffers even before the systolic pressure reaches critically low levels. Figure 16.5 presents typical tracings of arterial pressure that might be seen in the ICU in
a patient with progressive tamponade.

Fine points of cardiac auscultation are difficult to appreciate in a noisy, hectic trauma room. Usually, however, in patients with cardiac tamponade the heart sounds will
be very distant or even inaudible.

Jugular venous distention is easy to appreciate. It is important to remember that
straining and agitation or overtransfusion can cause jugular venous distention even
in a patient who does not have tamponade. It takes only minutes to pass a central venous pressure (CVP) line and in this way ascertain CVP precisely. (It is not even nec-

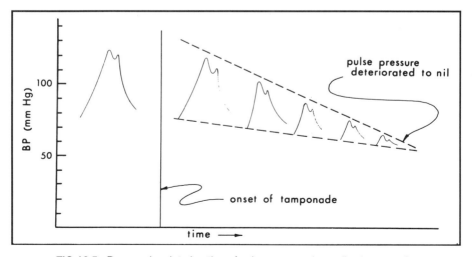

FIG.16.5. Progressive deterioration of pulse pressure in cardiac tamponade.

FIG.16.6. CXR in cardiac tamponade. Note the difference between normal left cardiac contour in **A** and loss of angle in left cardiac contour in CXR of patient in tamponade in **B**. In **B**, contour appears full and tense. (Reproduced with permission from Ref. 9.)

essary to use a manometer. The stopcock tubing will fill with blood when held upright in the air when the patient has tamponade.)

A word should be said about pulsus paradoxus and tamponade. Pulsus paradoxus refers to the inspiratory decrease in systolic blood pressure with breathing. A decrease of up to 15 mm Hg may be seen in normal subjects. Larger decreases are said to be characteristic of tamponade. To ascertain the degree of pulsus paradoxus requires excellent blood pressure-taking abilities and practice. The house officer should develop this skill. However, in the noisy emergency room, it may be difficult to ascertain the degree of paradox. It may be time-consuming also. Furthermore, a prominent pulsus paradoxus is an inconsistent finding in traumatic tamponade (5). For these reasons, with trauma, we rely less on determinations of pulsus paradoxus than we do in less acute circumstances. For example, in the setting of daily monitoring of chronic low-grade tamponade from uremic pericardial effusion on the medical ward, measuring pulsus paradoxus is indicated and useful.

A word should be said about the CXR in tamponade. The house officer often expects a large heart shadow in the patient with traumatic tamponade; this is not usually seen. The pericardium is largely inelastic; if it were elastic, tamponade would not occur. Although the pericardium, and the heart shadow, may grow tremendously with chronic effusions, with acute tamponade the usual finding is a normal heart shadow. Occasionally (Fig. 16.6), some straightening of the left heart border, obscuring the normal left pulmonary artery shadow, may be appreciated, giving the impression of "pressure" in the pericardial space.

Perhaps the most important point in diagnosis of tamponade is the patient's having sustained a penetrating injury in the region of the heart. If the patient has sustained a gunshot wound or knife wound near the heart and exhibits the classic triad of findings, chances are that he or she has tamponade. Keep in mind, however, that if the CVP is low in the hypotensive patient with chest trauma, the patient may well be hypovolemic without tamponade.

TREATMENT

Airway Obstruction

Injuries of the intrathoracic great airways can be devastating. Unlike upper-airway obstruction, where tracheostomy may provide airway access beyond the injury, tracheostomy is not useful with injuries to the intrathoracic trachea and mainstem bronchi. Rigid bronchoscopy is essential in diagnosis and treatment. If there is distortion and obstruction of the airway, it may be possible to advance the bronchoscope beyond the injury and thus to carry out positive pressure ventilation beyond the injury. The airway may be transected without distorting obstruction. In these cases, pleural and connective tissues may conduct the tidal volume, allowing effective spontaneous ventilation. If all continuity is lost, again the rigid bronchoscope may allow instrumentation and ventilation of the distal tracheobronchial tree. Surgery is required after initial respiratory support, though many patients with such injuries succumb before specialized care is available. **For the house officer the main task is prompt recognition of such injuries, so that the specialist can be called early.**

Flail Chest

Historically, flail chest has been treated by immobilization of the flail segment. This has been done by immobilizing in the "in" position (by sandbags or bricks) or in the "out" position (by grasping a rib with a towel clip attached to a weight hanging over a pulley). On occasion, internal fixation of rib fractures has been carried out surgically. This is fraught with difficulties and is usually unnecessary. **The modern treatment for flail chest is intubation and positive pressure ventilation.** When the lungs are expanded by positive pressure within the tracheobronchial tree, it makes no difference, physiologically, what the flail segment does. After 10 days to 2 weeks of ventilation, the chest wall begins to solidify, flailing diminishes, and the patient can be weaned to spontaneous ventilation and extubated.

Now, not every patient with flail chest requires intubation and positive pressure ventilation. Flails have different degrees of severity, and patients differ in the degree of embarrassment they can tolerate (i.e., the amount of ineffective tidal volume they can afford to lose). If a particular flail is well tolerated in a patient, without distress and without hypoventilation, no specific treatment is required. It is important to remember that elderly patients, especially, may initially tolerate the flail but tire progressively from the respiratory embarrassment. It is important that such patients be watched carefully over the first several days, both by clinical observation and by arterial blood gas measurements.

In recent years, increasing attention has been drawn to the fact that in flail chest significant pulmonary contusion more often than not accompanies the mechanical chest wall defect (6,7). It has been learned that the underlying contusion may be as important as the chest wall defect, and perhaps more so in certain cases. It has been shown that the contused lung is very sensitive to fluid administration; vigorous fluid and crystalloid administration by the trauma team can lead to pulmonary edema in the contused lung segments, with resultant hypoxia. Although avoidance of over-transfusion and "running the patient dry" are now accepted as important aspects of the care of patients with flail chest, most authorities would still agree that severe flails with respiratory embarrassment continue to require intubation and mechanical ventilation.

Sucking Chest Wound

The treatment for a sucking chest wound is an occlusive dressing. Vaseline gauze covered by sponges and tape works well. The occlusive dressing prevents the loss of tidal volume through the defect (the wasted ventilation of the pleural space discussed earlier in the section on physiology). Usually a closed (nontension) pneumothorax remains after placement of the occlusive dressing, but this does not represent a life-threatening condition. Astute medical technicians in battlefield circumstances have learned to have the injured patient with a sucking chest wound exhale fully immediately before placement of the occlusive dressing. This maneuver serves to minimize or eliminate residual pneumothorax. In the emergency room setting, a chest tube can be placed after application of the occlusive dressing to eliminate any residual pneumothorax.

Major chest wall defects will need eventually to be debrided and closed formally in the operating room. The treatment outlined earlier will prevent respiratory demise until formal treatment is undertaken.

Massive Hemothorax

House officers often consider placement of a chest tube to be the treatment for massive hemothorax. Although the chest tube is certainly helpful, it will be recalled from the earlier discussion that loss of ipsilateral lung function is not the key physiologic element in massive hemothorax. Rather, the key feature is **hypovolemia**—the patient exsanguinates. **Thus the treatment of massive hemothorax is volume replacement—specifically, administration of blood.** Although not usually critical, restoration of ipsilateral lung function by emptying the pleural space is also beneficial. Placement of a chest tube is therefore helpful and allows evaluation of the amount of blood lost and the ongoing rate of bleeding. The house officer should not be shocked if large amounts of blood are evacuated immediately. It is not uncommon for one drainage device to fill immediately. This volume usually represents blood already shed. The key criterion in further management is the ongoing rate of bleeding. **If bleeding continues at more than 200 ml/h for 3 h, operative intervention should be considered.** The specialist can address this question. The critical aspect of initial care by the house officer is volume replacement.

It is important to note that the **overwhelming majority of knife wounds of the lung and a large majority of gunshot wounds of the lung do not require surgical treatment.** The pulmonary arterial circuit is a low-pressure system. When the lung is expanded to the chest wall after tube placement, the irritated visceral and parietal pleural surfaces appose and adhere. Between the low pressures involved and the tamponading by apposed tissues, most pulmonary parenchymal injuries stop bleeding without exploration. Air leaks from the parenchyma can almost always be controlled by chest tube placement and apposition of pleural surfaces.

Tension Pneumothorax

The treatment for tension pneumothorax is chest tube placement. This is fairly straightforward. House officers often have heard of instrumenting the chest with a needle or plastic intravenous cannula. Although these maneuvers may occasionally be helpful, placement of a chest tube takes little more time and is far superior. Every house officer should know how to place a chest tube, as each will perform procedures that can be complicated by tension pneumothorax (especially thoracentesis and placement of central venous lines). Key concepts regarding chest tubes are covered in Chapter 17.

Cardiac Tamponade

The management of cardiac tamponade is not as straightforward. It is useful to consider first the *medical* treatment of tamponade, that is, treatment without needles, tubes, and surgery. We will, for the moment, "tie the surgeon's hands." Here the mechanism by which tamponade hurts the heart must be remembered. In tamponade, the heart cannot pump because the heart cannot fill. To get the heart to pump, one must get it to fill. To get the heart to fill, one must provide a gradient from the cavae to the RV. As the RV pressures are high from pressure transmitted from the pericardial space, CVP must be raised quite high. **Thus the medical treatment of tamponade is volume administration** (5). The house officer should be cautioned that nurses and inexperienced physicians may look skeptically on giving volume to a patient whose CVP is already high. When blood pressure is failing in tamponade, one must drive the CVP as high as possible to fill the heart and get the heart to pump. Pulmonary edema is not an issue. Blood is not even reaching the left heart, let alone backing up in the pulmonary circuit. Acute right-sided CVP elevation is not dangerous. Were it to continue, edema, ascites, and hepatic engorgement might develop, but with acute tamponade and shock, the patient's life is at stake and a brief elevation of CVP is a small price to pay. Often crystalloid replacement to drive CVP up is successful in restoring some effective circulation in tamponade.

Inotropes are not part of the usual treatment of tamponade because they do not address the underlying physiology, which is failure of the heart to fill. Further, young patients in shock probably will have great release of endogenous catecholamines. Nevertheless, in desperate circumstances, inotropic support can be instituted. Although β-agonism is probably unnecessary, some α-agonism may raise systemic pressures, albeit at the expense of organ perfusion, and allow better coronary perfusion. This could improve cardiac performance.

Patients who develop tamponade after cardiac surgery may not have the healthy heart of the young traumatized patient. These patients may benefit from inotropic support before mechanical correction of postoperative tamponade is achieved.

The medical interventions discussed are important, but they represent essentially temporizing measures; the defect in tamponade is a mechanical one that requires a mechanical correction. We will discuss now what can be done after the surgeon's hands are "untied."

Pericardiocentesis is the first step in the surgical management of acute traumatic tamponade. The subxyphoid approach is illustrated in Fig. 16.7. As is well appreciated, because of the inelastic nature of the pericardium, removal of even a small volume of blood can significantly lower intrapericardial pressures and produce

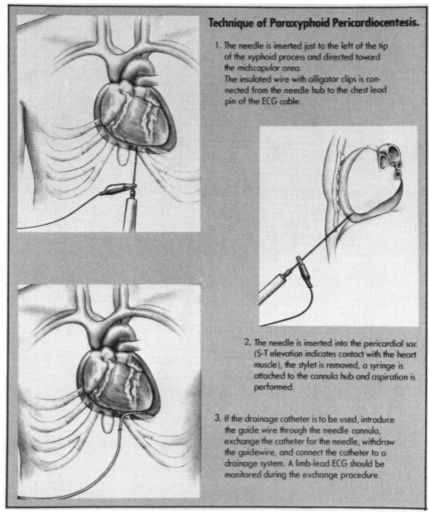

Technique of Paraxyphoid Pericardiocentesis.

1. The needle is inserted just to the left of the tip of the xyphoid process and directed toward the midscapular area.
   The insulated wire with alligator clips is connected from the needle hub to the chest lead pin of the ECG cable.

2. The needle is inserted into the pericardial sac (S-T elevation indicates contact with the heart muscle), the stylet is removed, a syringe is attached to the cannula hub and aspiration is performed.

3. If the drainage catheter is to be used, introduce the guide wire through the needle cannula, exchange the catheter for the needle, withdraw the guidewire, and connect the catheter to a drainage system. A limb-lead ECG should be monitored during the exchange procedure.

FIG.16.7. Subxyphoid pericardiocentesis. The needle is shown connected to a V lead of the ECG, for detection of contact with the surface of the heart. (Reproduced with permission of Mansfield Scientific, Inc.)

dramatic improvement in vital signs. Pericardiocentesis in this setting is not easy and not always effective. Blood is likely to be thick and partially clotted; it may not draw back through the needle. The heart, coronary arteries, lungs, and liver may be injured.

Most authorities agree that a patient who requires pericardiocentesis for acute traumatic tamponade should be taken for operation to control the injury. The alternative—waiting to see if bleeding recurs—represents an unnecessary and possibly dangerous delay that is unlikely to prevent surgery.

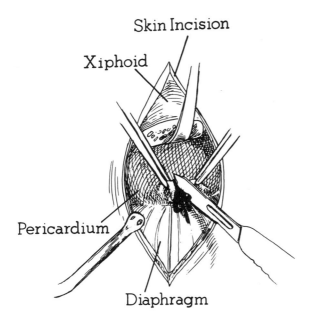

Skin Incision

Xiphoid

Pericardium

Diaphragm

FIG.16.8. Subxyphoid pericardiotomy. (Reprinted with permission from Ref. 10.)

The house officer should be familiar with another technique that is available for decompressing the pericardium urgently. This is **subxyphoid pericardiotomy** (Fig. 16.8). This procedure can be done on the emergency ward or in the operating room under local anesthesia (or without anesthesia if vital signs are failing). If vital signs are preserved, this procedure may be performed to prevent the deterioration seen with induction of general anesthesia. The procedure is done by making a midline vertical incision over the lower sternum and the xyphoid process, excising the xyphoid process, and spreading the few intervening diaphragmatic fibers to visualize the pericardium. Then one picks up the pericardium and incises it. This provides immediate, thorough decompression of the pericardial space. A condition of tamponade can be converted in this way to a condition of cardiac injury without tamponade. Once this is performed, the patient will not die of tamponade. However, bleeding may be vigorous. With hemodynamic stability restored by the pericardiotomy, sternotomy or thoracotomy can then be done for definitive control of the injury.

In a postoperative patient who develops tamponade, opening the lower end of the wound and removing the sutures from the linea alba provides similar relief of tamponade under urgent circumstances (see Fig. 15.2). Formal exploration and reclosure usually follow.

ADDITIONAL TOPIC: SYSTEMIC AIR EMBOLISM

The house officer must be familiar with the fascinating phenomenon of **systemic air embolism** following parenchymal lung injuries (8). The pathophysiology of this condition is as follows (Fig. 16.9). A parenchymal lung injury disrupts both *bronchi* and *pulmonary veins*. Air from the disrupted bronchi can enter the open pulmonary veins. (This is especially likely to occur if the trauma patient is on positive pressure ventilation. It is also especially likely if the patient is hypovolemic, as is often the case in major trauma. The positive pressure ventilation makes the air exiting the bronchi more likely to find routes of egress—into the pulmonary veins. The hypovolemia leads to lower pressure in the pulmonary veins—so that, instead of bleeding, these veins suck air liberated from the bronchi.) From the pulmonary veins, the air is carried into the left atrium, and from there to the left ventricle. From the left ventri-

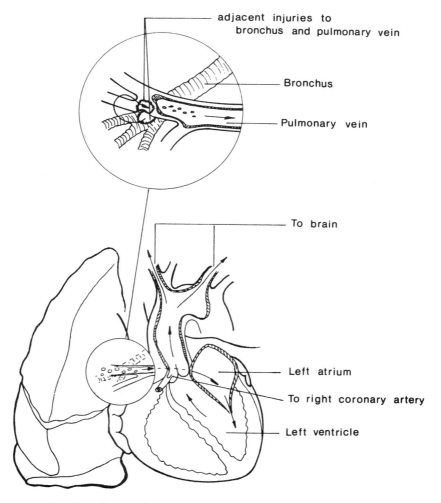

FIG. 16.9. Schematic representation of systemic air embolism. (See text.)

cle, the air is ejected into the aorta and the systemic arterial tree, where it can cause ischemia by virtue of "air lock" in a specific vascular bed. If this air travels to the brain, it can cause a stroke. If it travels to the heart, it causes myocardial ischemia, often with cardiac arrest from ventricular fibrillation.

A common scenario is that the patient with a parenchymal lung injury, either stab or gunshot, enters the trauma room hypotensive, hypoxic, and agitated. On spontaneous ventilation, the pressure relationships do not produce air embolism. The patient is intubated for stabilization, and promptly arrests. The cause is often systemic air embolism. The institution of positive pressure ventilation has forced the air out of the bronchi and into the pulmonary veins. The right coronary artery, located just at the origin of the aorta, and directly anteriorly, where the air bubble tends to go by gravity, "traps" the bubble, leading to myocardial ischemia and ventricular fibrillation.

Systemic air embolism can be seen also with iatrogenic trauma, as is needle biopsy of the lung, chest tube placement, and forceful irrigation of empyema tubes.

The house officer must maintain a high index of suspicion for systemic air embolism in traumatic chest injury. Air embolism is overwhelmingly underdiagnosed. The treatment is urgent thoracotomy. The patient is placed in Trendelenburg position to direct air away from the brain. The bronchovenous connection is interrupted by clamping the site of parenchymal injury or the hilum of the lung. Air is vented from the aorta and the left ventricular apex. Open resuscitation is carried out. Formal lung resection is performed once hemodynamic stability is restored. Although systemic air embolism is almost invariably fatal, occasional survival with urgent thoracotomy has been obtained. Such thoracotomy must, of course, be carried out only by properly trained personnel. The house officer on duty needs to be aware of the syndrome and to have a high index of suspicion—so that he obtains the expert backup required.

The house officer can help to prevent systemic air embolism by carrying out volume repletion before intubation. Avoiding high inspiratory pressures is also of benefit.

The phenomenon of *systemic* air embolism discussed here is to be contrasted with *venous* air embolism, in which air entering the great veins, usually from an open central line, travels to the lungs, causing an airlock in the pulmonary arteries with attendant cadiopulmonary collapse.

ADDITIONAL POINTS

Although specifics of operative repair of particular cardiac and pulmonary injuries are beyond the scope of this text, a number additional general guidelines (8) deserve mention.

- **Stab wounds anywhere in the "thoracic mantle"** (see Fig. 16.10) **should be suspected of producing cardiac injury.**

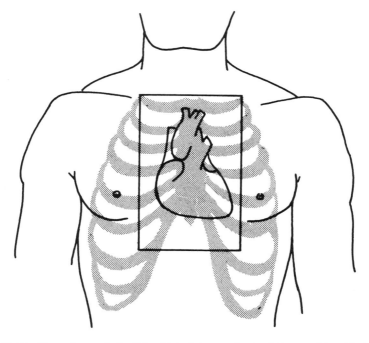

FIG. 16.10. The "thoracic mantle," within which stab wounds should be considered to have produced cardiac injury until proven otherwise. (Adapted with permission from Ref. 11.)

- **Gunshot wounds anywhere in the vicinity of the chest should always be suspected of producing cardiac injury**, because of the unpredictable trajectory of bullets in the body.
- **Finger control can stop bleeding from most wounds of the atria, ventricles, and aorta.** Application of clamps and instruments urgently under suboptimal circumstances is usually not necessary and can cause severe injury.
- **Because of the high position of the diaphragms in expiration, injuries anywhere below the nipples may produce intra-abdominal as well as intrathoracic injury.**
- **Emergency room thoracotomy is indicated only for *penetrating* cardiac injuries in patients *in extremis*** (without preserved blood pressure). For *blunt* injury, the dismal yield in survival does not justify emergency room thoracotomy. For patients with penetrating injury, especially when they present with sinus rhythm despite absent blood pressure, emergency room thoracotomy is not infrequently life-saving. For patients with preserved, albeit severely depressed, blood pressure, a trip to the operating room—with its better lighting and instrumentation—is much better than the difficult and dangerous emergency room thoracotomy.
- **The approach to transmediastinal gunshot wounds does not always mandate surgery.** If vital signs are unstable, immediate exploration is indeed required. If

the patient is entirely stable, as is often the case, specialized, systematic evaluation of organs at risk may at times suffice. It is surprising how often the "educated" bullet traverses the mediastinum without producing major injury. Aortography is essential to rule out great vessel arterial injury. (There is no need to do any diagnostic studies to rule out occult venous injuries. If a venous injury is not actively bleeding, it will heal on its own.) Esophagography is essential to rule out esophageal injury. Bronchoscopy is essential to rule out central bronchial injury.

Subxyphoid pericardial window (see earlier) can rule out intrapericardial bleeding. Cardiac echo may provide similar confirmation that there is no bloody pericardial effusion. Careful ICU observation, especially with echocardiographic exam, may suffice in place of pericardial window in selected patients.

If the house officer keeps the basic physiology of these few categories of dysfunction after chest trauma in mind and adheres to the treatment guidelines outlined, he or she can be assured of satisfactory early management of thoracic and cardiac injuries.

REFERENCES

1. Rutherford R. Thoracic injuries. In: Ballinger W, Rutherford R, Zuidema G, eds. *The management of trauma.* Philadelphia: WB Saunders; 1973:333–395.
2. Hood M. Trauma to the chest. In: Sabiston D, Spencer F, eds. *Surgery of the chest.* Philadelphia: WB Saunders; 1983:291–317.
3. Symbas P. *Traumatic injuries of the heart and great vessels.* Springfield, IL: Charles C Thomas; 1972.
4. Trauma. In: Shoemaker W, Thompson W, Holbrook P, eds. *Textbook of critical care.* Philadelphia: WB Saunders; 1984:891–898.
5. Shoemaker W. Pericardial tamponade. In: Shoemaker W, Thompson W, Holbrook P, eds. *Textbook of critical care.* Philadelphia: WB Saunders; 1984:493–497.
6. Trinkle J, Richardson J, Franz J, et al. Management of flail chest without mechanical ventilation. *Ann Thorac Surg* 1975;19:355–363.
7. Shackford S, Virgilio R, Peters R. Selective use of ventilator therapy in flail chest injury. *J Thorac Cardiovasc Surg* 1981;81:194–201.
8. Elefteriades JA. Chest trauma. In: Kreis DJ, Gomez GA, eds. *Trauma management.* Boston: Little, Brown; 1989.
9. Thompson T. *Primer of clinical radiology.* Boston: Little, Brown;1980.
10. Sabiston DC, Jr., Spencer FC. *Gibbon's surgery of the chest*, 7th edition. Philadelphia: WB Saunders;1974.
11. Karrel R, Shaffer MA, Franaszek JB. Emergency diagnosis, resuscitation, and treatment of acute penetrating cardiac trauma. *Ann Emerg Med* 1982;11:504

SUGGESTED FURTHER READING

Rutherford, R. Thoracic injuries. In: Ballinger W, Rutherford R, Zuidema G, eds. *The management of trauma.* Philadelphia: WB Saunders; 1973:333–395.

A particularly lucid account, at just the right level of sophistication for the interested house officer. Lists the six devastating conditions discussed in this chapter.

Shoemaker W. Pericardial tamponade. In: Shoemaker W, Thompson W, Holbrook P, eds. *Textbook of critical care.* Philadelphia: WB Saunders; 1984:493–497.

A concise and clear account of this important condition.

17 Chest Tubes

Junior house officers commonly require instruction on a number of aspects of chest tube use and care. Patients routinely come to the ICU from cardiac or thoracic surgery with chest tubes in place. Not infrequently, additional tubes may be required during the patient's ICU stay, for pneumothorax or hemothorax. The house officer must be comfortable with all aspects of chest tube placement and care in order to avoid errors in patient management.

TUBE VARIABLES: SITE, TECHNIQUE, MATERIAL, SIZE

A question that often arises is where to place the tube. **In general, it is usually recommended that a tube placed for pneumothorax be directed anteriorly and superiorly and that a tube placed for hemothorax be directed posteriorly and inferiorly**; these sites are selected because air rises anteriorly and fluid falls posteriorly in a supine patient. The anatomic guidelines for anterior and posterior tube placement are depicted in Fig. 17.1. The anterior site of choice is the midclavicular line in the second or third intercostal space. (The angle of Louis marks the second intercostal space.) A tube placed more medially endangers the great vessels. A tube placed more cephalad endangers the subclavian artery and vein. A tube placed more caudad endangers the pulmonary hilum. The second or third interspace in the midclavicular line is uniformly and widely safe. The posterior site of choice is the midaxillary line in

207

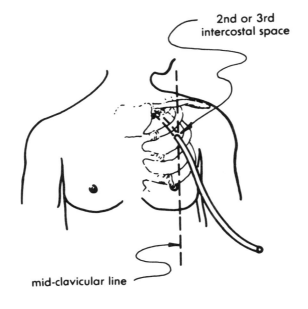

2nd or 3rd
intercostal space

mid-clavicular line

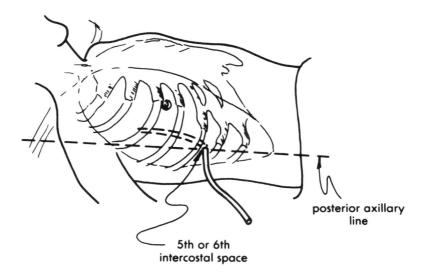

posterior axillary
line

5th or 6th
intercostal space

FIG. 17.1. Standard sites for anterior (top) and lateral (bottom) chest tube placement.

the fifth or sixth intercostal space. (Two finger breadths below the nipple will approximate this level.) To place the tube more posteriorly would cause the supine patient to lie on the tube; this is uncomfortable and may kink or occlude the tube. To place the tube more caudad risks injury to the diaphragm and abdominal structures. The diaphragm, it will be recalled, can rise anteriorly almost to the nipple line during expiration. Furthermore, the costodiaphragmatic sulcus, the space of safety between the chest wall and the diaphragm, narrows quickly as one proceeds caudad.

Despite the preceding guidelines, in actual fact, **in the virgin chest**—without prior surgery or inflammatory adhesions, and with a free pleural space—**a tube placed at any site will evacuate air or fluid effectively**. The midaxillary line approach, especially, is universally applicable for air or fluid.

When the pleural space is not free—that is, when there exist adhesions from prior surgery, trauma, or inflammation—tube placement must be selected carefully. This will usually require the guidance of an experienced chest surgeon. If a pneumothorax occurs in a free chest, the lung comes down from the chest wall symmetrically along its perimeter. If a region of lung does not come down symmetrically, this suggests a tethering to the chest wall by adhesions (Fig. 17.2). Fluid in a free chest forms a meniscus between the lung and the chest wall, giving a characteristic chest x-ray (CXR) appearance (Fig. 17.3). A localized fluid shadow implies that the fluid is loculated in a scarred pleural space. A nonuniform contour of a pneumothorax or loculation of a hemothorax should raise a red flag for the house officer. To place a tube by rote in standard fashion (anteriorly or in the posterior axillary line) in a pleural space with adhesions risks injury to adherent underlying lung. The site for placement must be selected carefully on the basis of three-dimensional reconstruction of the anatomy, using posteroanterior and lateral CXRs or even a CT scan. The house officer may be best off studying the anatomy in detail, selecting a site, and then placing a radiopaque marker (a paper clip works well) at that site. Repeat two-dimensional x-rays will confirm appropriate selection of the proposed tube site or suggest adjustment of selection. **Above all, a tube must not be placed unless there is an underlying space, either air or fluid, at that site.** Several times yearly on a busy chest service, a tube is forcefully placed into the parenchyma of the lung because these important points are not appreciated.

Another frequent question is whether the tube should be placed via a trocar or by following a tract created by blunt finger dissection and a Kelly clamp. The house officer should gain experience with each method under careful bedside supervision. Although the trocar system may allow the experienced surgeon more accurate direction of a smaller tube into complex pleural spaces, the blunt, Kelly clamp approach is more widely useful for the house officer, as the large-bore tubes required for trauma and postoperatively can be placed only by this means.

The patient will feel pain when air or fluid is removed from the pleural space after tube placement. The pain of which the patient complains, although worrisome, usually signifies the approximation of visceral and parietal pleurae that is the desired end result of evacuation of air or fluid from the pleural space.

FIG. 17.2. Chest x-ray in free (**A**) and nonfree (**B**) pneumothorax. In **A** pneumothorax is on patient's left. In **B** pneumothorax is at base and at apex on patient's right. In nonfree pneumothorax, tethering of the lung to the chest wall prevents uniform symmetrical collapse. (**A** is reprinted with permission from Ref. 1.)

FIG. 17.3. Chest x-ray in free (**A**) and loculated (**B**) pleural effusion. Loculated effusion is contained in one area against the chest wall. (**B** is reprinted with permission from Ref. 1.)

Tube type and size must be selected. Three major materials may be chosen: rubber, plastic, or silicone (Silastic). Red rubber tubes are soft and pliable and come in small sizes. Some surgeons feel that these tubes are preferable because they irritate the pleura and cause the sticking together of the visceral and parietal layers that is so often desired (as in pneumothorax). A disadvantage of the red rubber tubes is that they tend to obstruct easily and quickly with clot or fibrin. Another disadvantage is that many of the rubber tubes are not radiopaque; this may confound assessment of placement by CXR. Clear plastic tubes are very resistant to clotting. These tubes come in the large sizes necessary postoperatively or for trauma. The plastic tubes, moreover, always incorporate radiopaque markers. For the house officer, a plastic rather than a rubber tube is probably the better choice. Silicone tubes are even more resistant to occlusion by clot or fibrin (this almost never occurs) and have become very popular for use at the time of open-heart surgery.

House officers frequently select a tube too large or too small for the intended purpose. Large tubes are more difficult to place and more uncomfortable for the patient. Small tubes cannot handle heavy drainage of thick material. Some general guidelines for selection are as follows. The patient with a spontaneous pneumothorax and only air in the pleural space needs only a small tube: a 16F is excellent for this purpose. This tube will not be too uncomfortable to place but can be relied upon to evacuate air as long as required. For trauma or for a frank postoperative hemothorax, a 32F tube is appropriate. Even clots pass well through a tube this large. For an effusion that is not frankly bloody, an intermediate size, say 24F or 26F, is appropriate. A tube this size will properly drain an effusion, even a thick one, without entailing severe discomfort during placement.

DRAINAGE SYSTEMS: BOTTLE SYSTEMS AND DISPOSABLE DRAINAGE UNITS

The end of the chest tube cannot be left open to air, because atmospheric pressure in the pleural cavity would cause pneumothorax. Various drainage systems are available, from simple to complex. These will be reviewed in some detail, for misconceptions abound and errors are frequent.

The Heimlich Valve

Perhaps the simplest drainage system is the Heimlich valve (Fig. 17.4). This is a rubber flutter valve that allows only unidirectional movement of air and fluid (out of the chest). Care should be taken to insert the valve in the proper direction. Air or fluid can force the rubber leaflets apart for egress from the chest. When egress has occurred, the rubber leaflets approximate, preventing entry of air into the chest. Inspiration further approximates the leaflets, maintaining negative intrathoracic pressure.

This simple device can be very useful under emergency circumstances, such as on the battlefield. Under such circumstances, this device can allow treatment of pneu-

FIG. 17.4. The Heimlich valve.

mo- or hemothorax without complex equipment. However, the device itself is messy, as no collection system is incorporated. Furthermore, monitoring air or fluid leak is difficult. In the hospital, other devices are more useful.

Bottle Systems

The **one-bottle system** represents the next level of sophistication above the Heimlich valve (Fig. 17.5). In this system, a length of tubing connects the chest tube itself to a glass or plastic straw passing through a stopper into a large glass bottle. Another glass rod vents the inside of the bottle to air. Sterile water is added to a level of several centimeters above the end of the drainage straw. This level provides the so-called water seal.

from patient

open to air

Water-seal Bottle

FIG. 17.5. The one-bottle system.

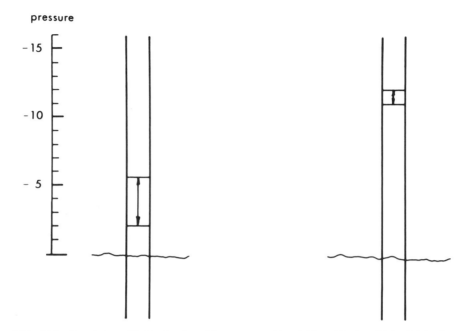

FIG. 17.6. Respiratory tidal fluctuation of the water seal level. The wide, low tidal at left is characteristic of the early period following thoracotomy. The narrow, high tidal at right is characteristic of the late period following thoracotomy, indicating sealing of pleural space.

Air and fluid can still drain easily from the pleural space with the tip submerged. However, the pleural space remains sealed, as air cannot enter the submerged tip of the straw. With inspiration, water may be lifted several centimeters up the straw, but no air can enter.

This simple system is remarkably versatile and effective. Almost any thoracic operation can be accommodated by this one-bottle system. Indeed, this very system is still preferred at some thoracic centers.

Fluid drainage can be monitored by graduating the bottle and marking on a tape along its side. Subtracting the original amount of fluid used for water seal from the total contents at a particular time gives the amount of fluid drained.

An air leak is easily detected: Bubbles are seen exiting from the drainage straw. The greater the bubbling, the greater the air leak from the chest.

The drainage straw acts as a manometer, allowing continuous, instantaneous monitoring of intrapleural pressure. With inspiration, water is drawn up into the tube. The height of water drawn above the level in the bottle equals, in centimeters of water, the negative pressure in the chest. When an air leak exists, water is drawn up only with inspiration. As the air leak seals, negative pressure supervenes throughout the respiratory cycle. (It will be recalled from physiology that a negative inspiratory pressure of 10–15 cm H_2O normally exists in the pleural space.) **As the pulmonary**

parenchyma seals more effectively with time after a thoracic operation, the water column rises higher in the straw. The one-bottle system provides the surgeon all this information about intrathoracic events.

The concept of tidal fluctuation is important as well. When a chest tube is first placed, the level of water in the drainage straw fluctuates widely with each breath (Fig. 17.6); this fluctuation is called the *respiratory tidal.* The overall height of the water level rises with parenchymal sealing as time passes after a thoracic operation; also, **with time, the respiratory tidal decreases.** This reflects apposition and sticking of visceral and parietal pleurae around the tube, excluding it from free communication with the pleural space. This occurs only as the leakage of fluid and air abates; it is a good sign, indicating that tubes can be removed soon. All this additional information about intrathoracic events is provided as well by the water seal manometer in the one-bottle system. Assessment of these events becomes second nature with experience.

The one-bottle system does have a disadvantage: Because effluent fluid collects in the bottle, the water level rises with time. The rising level provides a stronger water seal, for intrapleural air must reach a higher pressure before it bubbles through and is evacuated. If the fluid level is allowed to rise unchecked, a pneumothorax may result.

FIG. 17.7. The two-bottle system.

FIG. 17.8. The three-bottle system.

It is best to change the bottle at intervals to maintain a water seal only 2–3 cm in height.

The **two-bottle system** (Fig. 17.7) adds a collecting bottle in series between the patient and the water seal bottle. Function is entirely identical except that the interposed collection bottle prevents the undesired rise in water seal height as drainage collects. Fluctuations in the water seal straw have exactly the same significance as with the one-bottle system.

The **three-bottle system** adds one more elaboration (Fig. 17.8). The vent of the water seal bottle is connected to suction, but via a third, suction control bottle. (Suction could be applied directly to the water seal bottle vent if accurately controlled suction were available; this is not usually the case.) Because hospital wall suction is excessively strong and can cause significant tissue injury, a foolproof suction control is mandatory. This foolproof control is provided by the third bottle. The vent of the water seal bottle is connected to a straw passing into the suction control bottle. Another straw passes out of the suction control bottle to the wall suction. A third straw passes into the bottle with its tip resting below an adjustable level of water. The level of water is specified by the physician. This level limits the suction applied to the chest tube. For example, if 15 cm of saline is placed in the bottle, negative pressure applied will be 15 cm regardless of the amount of wall suction applied. Any wall negative pressure greater than 15 cm will merely draw air in through the open straw. The third

FIG. 17.9. A commonly used disposable collection system. (Reproduced with permission of Deknatel, Inc.)

bottle should always be bubbling; otherwise less than the specified amount of suction is being applied from the wall. The house officer must recognize that this bubbling represents not an air leak but just suction control. Air leak, as with the one- and two-bottle systems, is read only in the water seal bottle. The simple addition of this third bottle eliminates the danger of parenchymal injury from excess wall suction.

Disposable Systems

A variety of disposable systems, which house an entire three-bottle system in one plastic enclosure, are available (Fig. 17.9). The house officer should recognize that these disposable units are just a three-bottle system in a compact, convenient, disposable, nonbreakable configuration. Each has a collection, a water seal, and a suction control chamber. The house officer should become familiar with the particular disposable system used at his or her hospital and identify each of the three key elements. In the water seal chamber, air leak, pleural pressure level, and respiratory tidal can be followed and carry the same meaning as in the bottle systems. In the suction control chamber, a variable amount of fluid can be added to achieve a specified level of suction. As in the three-bottle system, the suction control chamber should always be bubbling.

MANAGEMENT PARTICULARS

Suction or Water Seal

Although suction is used routinely at many centers, **almost all patients can be handled perfectly well with simple water seal.** For almost all patients, application of suction is superfluous. Even a major pneumothorax can be evacuated through water seal in just a few respiratory cycles. Even the moderate air leaks that follow lobectomy are easily handled by simple water seal. Only those patients with massive air leak require suction; **suction does remove air more effectively than water seal when the leak is massive.** Inadequacy of water seal to relieve pneumothorax completely will be apparent from incomplete expansion of the lung on the CXR obtained after lobectomy or following tube placement for spontaneous or traumatic pneumothorax. The remaining rim of air can be evacuated by addition of suction to the system.

Nonetheless, at most hospitals, suction is used routinely. Though not strictly necessary in most cases, it is not at all detrimental. The house officer can usually expect to see this policy unless he or she specifies otherwise.

Clamping of Tubes

Despite common misconceptions, with one exception, **chest tubes and apparatus should never be clamped**. Nursing protocols at many hospitals have perpetuated the myth that during transport the patient's chest tube system should be clamped. This offers no benefit and may be dangerous for the patient with an ongoing air leak. With the system clamped, the patient with an air leak may develop a tension pneumothorax. **The proper state for transport of a chest tube patient is water seal.** On water seal, no tension pneumothorax can develop; rather, air under pressure in the pleural space will drain freely through the water seal.

The one exception to the rule not to clamp is during evaluation in preparation for tube removal (see below).

Suction Control

Despite common misconceptions, **increasing the amount of wall suction, to increase bubbling in the suction control chamber, does not increase effectiveness of the pleural drainage system**; this merely serves to draw more atmospheric air through the suction control water level and to cause more noise. **The proper way to increase effective suction is to add water to the suction control chamber.** This transmits more of the wall suction to the patient before entraining atmospheric air. Usually 15–20 cm H_2O is used routinely. When required, this can be increased to 25–30 cm H_2O.

In *very* rare cases, multiple tubes attached to multiple suction devices may be required to accommodate the most massive air leaks. In this case, surgical control of the bronchial or parenchymal defect may be required.

Assessment of Severity of Air Leak

The severity of air leak an be evaluated by the amount of bubbling in the water seal chamber of the chest drainage apparatus. In particular, **the severity of the air leak is reflected by the proportion of the respiratory cycle during which bubbling occurs**. In the spontaneously respiring patient, a mild air leak will cause bubbling during peak expiration only; it is during expiration that airway pressures are maximal. With a moderate leak, bubbling occupies the entire expiratory phase. With a severe air leak, bubbling occurs during the inspiratory phase as well as during all of the expiratory phase. With massive leaks, bubbling is continuous.

In patients on positive pressure ventilation, these relationships are reversed. A mild leak expresses itself as bubbling during inspiration; on the ventilator, inspiration is a positive pressure phenomenon. During expiration, bubbling ceases except with more severe leaks.

The house officer should recognize that **air leak is normal following major pulmonary resections**; it does *not* imply surgical error. Rather, leak is expected from all areas where lung parenchyma is divided, especially at sites of incomplete fissures. As explained in Chapter 19, these parenchymal leaks uniformly stop within a day or two of pleural apposition.

The question often arises whether an air leak is actually coming from the patient or from a leak in the tubing system. If the tubing and connections between the patient and the drainage device are not tight, air can enter the system, giving the spurious appearance of an air leak. This question can be resolved in a straightforward manner. Finding a continuous leak, without significant variation in bubbling with the respiratory cycle, serves as a clue that air may be entering the system. (Only very large true air leaks would show this pattern.) The question is resolved by temporarily clamping the chest tube at the patient's chest wall. If the leak is false (i.e., caused by air entering the system from outside), bubbling continues. If the leak is true (i.e., coming from the patient), bubbling ceases. When a false leak is confirmed, connections and tubing are examined and defects corrected. When true leak is confirmed, drainage is resumed as previously.

Occasionally, the defect causing a false leak may be not in the tubing system but between the chest tube proper and the patient's chest wall. In this circumstance, the suction in the apparatus draws air into the chest (between the tube and its tract in the chest wall) and then evacuates it through the tube. Disappearance of the leak on water seal may suggest this circumstance. Confirmation is provided when the leak disappears permanently with placement of an occlusive pursestring suture or occlusive Vaseline gauze dressing around the tube entrance site.

Tubing Care

The rubber tubing that connects the chest tube to the drainage device is frequently improperly or inadequately managed, especially on wards that handle chest tubes infrequently. Often the tubing is found occluded by the patient's own weight. In the presence of a significant air leak, of course, this can cause a tension pneumothorax. A less blatant but more common error is to allow a loop in the tubing (Fig. 17.10). If water collects in the loop to a height greater than the suction control limit (usually set at 15–20 cm H_2O), the tube will be effectively sealed—just as if it were clamped! This also can cause pneumothorax and tension pneumothorax. **The tubing from patient to drainage device must always remain horizontal or descending, never ascending or looping.** A level, horizontal loop that lies flat on the mattress is permissible.

Also, in general, the tubing and drainage device should not be raised above the patient's level, for reverse drainage is possible.

Stripping of Tubes

Some surgeons and some ICUs practice stripping of tubes. Some use the powdered hand or even a mechanical device for this purpose. Others feel that stripping can promote bleeding. It has, in fact, been demonstrated experimentally that stripping can produce very high negative pressures in the chest. These negative pressures could dislodge normal, useful clots at potential bleeding sites. Institutional policies vary, but we prefer "walking" the drainage fluid through the tube rather than forceful stripping.

incorrect

correct

FIG. 17.10. An ascending segment of tubing or loops in the tubing (top) leading to the collection bottle will cause a fluid trap that disables the system. The proper method is to keep the tubing always level or descending (bottom).

Tube Removal

In general, **mediastinal chest tubes placed following cardiac surgery can be removed when drainage falls to less than 100 ml over 8 h.** When this criterion is met, the chance of significant subsequent accumulation of blood or fluid is remote. This criterion is usually met by the morning of the second day after surgery.

For tubes placed following pulmonary surgery, both air and fluid drainage criteria must be met. Most surgeons insist on leaving tubes in place at least 24 or 48 h beyond the last time that any air leak was noted. The reason for this delay is to allow continued strong apposition of visceral and parietal pleurae under the influence of suction to achieve secure "sticking" of these layers. Following noncardiac chest surgery, the fluid criterion is somewhat more stringent than following cardiac surgery: Most surgeons will not remove tubes until drainage is less than 100 or 150 ml/24 h. The intent is to minimize the likelihood of accumulation of a significant postoperative pleural effusion. These criteria are to some extent traditional and arbitrary. Recent studies suggest that the traditional criteria may be too conservative.

Occasionally, the presence of the tube itself can promote serous drainage. In this case, the experienced chest surgeon may make the decision to remove tubes despite drainage that exceeds the preceding criteria.

For tubes placed following spontaneous pneumothorax, as for tubes placed after pulmonary surgery, it is customary to allow 24 or 48 h beyond the last noted air leak for optimal seal. Occasionally, we will clamp the tube for several hours prior to anticipated removal when we want to rule out intermittent bubbling. This low level of leak may not be detectable even with frequent monitoring of the water seal chamber. With the tube clamped, however, even a small leak will manifest a pneumothorax within several hours on CXR. If no pneumothorax is realized, intermittent bubbling has been ruled out, and the tube may safely be removed.

When a tube is removed, the tract must be sealed in some way until the body tissues close. The body's own seal is usually complete within 48 h. Until that time, two alternatives are available. Some surgeons place a pursestring, or "U," stitch around the chest tube site; this is in addition to the securing stitch and is tightened as the tube is withdrawn. Alternatively, a Vaseline gauze and dry sponge dressing may be taped tightly in place over the opening as the tube is withdrawn. This dressing can be removed in 48 h.

In spontaneously respiring patients, tubes are withdrawn during forced expiration; this prevents air entry into the chest. **In patients on mechanical ventilation, tubes are withdrawn during positive pressure inspiration,** for the same reason. In either setting, tubes must be pulled sharply and quickly, to prevent air entry. A safe rule is that when multiple tubes are present and attached to the same drainage device, they may be clamped, cut, and removed separately.

The house officer usually obtains a CXR after tube removal to ascertain that no air has been let into the chest. When tubes are purely mediastinal, as following cardiac surgery, this is probably unnecessary. Even with cardiac surgery, however, tubes may be placed in the pleural space if the pleura is entered during the operative procedure. Unless the house officer is certain that tubes are exclusively mediastinal, not pleural, it is best to obtain a CXR. Again, local custom will dictate.

The house officer should realize that even if air is let in during tube removal, there is no need to panic. This air has come from the outside, not from the bronchial tree or the lung parenchyma. There is no reason to expect a worsening of the pneumothorax. Rather, with time, spontaneous resolution will occur. The house officer should review the CXR with more senior personnel to determine if the iatrogenic pneumothorax is small enough to be tolerated by the patient until spontaneous resolution; if not, another tube will need to be placed.

SUBCUTANEOUS, CERVICAL, AND MEDIASTINAL EMPHYSEMA

Subcutaneous emphysema, with its characteristic "bubbly" sensation on palpation, may occur when a pneumothorax decompresses itself into the soft tissues (as via a chest wall injury or a chest tube site). This can be seen especially when the pleural space is obliterated by prior surgery or inflammation, so that the lung parenchyma leaks air but cannot fall away from the chest wall. This condition can progress rapidly but, though unsightly, is not dangerous. If an intrapleural air space exists, a chest tube should be placed and will prevent further accumulation. If subcutaneous emphysema has become massive or threatens to do so, small skin incisions can be made infraclavicularly, with spreading of soft tissues by clamp. Regular "milking" of subcutaneous air through the incisions by the nurses will permit early resolution.

Cervical emphysema—and its radiographic counterpart, mediastinal emphysema—can be seen whenever a parenchymal leak dissects along the bronchial tree into the mediastinum. Injury to the bronchus itself is occasionally the cause. (See Chapter 16.) Cervical and mediastinal emphysema are rarely of physiologic importance. In rare cases, when great pressure develops, a tamponade-like effect on the heart may occur. If deterioration in vital signs is felt to be occurring on this basis, total decompression can be obtained by performing an "almost tracheostomy" (2). Dissection is carried out as for tracheostomy, but the trachea itself is not opened. This vents all cervical continuations of the mediastinal tissue planes, decompresses the heart, and restores vital signs.

By understanding these guidelines, modifying them according to local practice, and gaining some hands-on experience, the house officer should become comfortably capable in chest tube management.

REFERENCES

1. Sutton D. *Radiology and imaging for medical students*, 4th edition. New York: Churchill Livingston; 1982.
2. Von Hippel A. *Chest tubes and chest bottles.* Springfield, IL: Charles C Thomas; 1970.

SUGGESTED FURTHER READING

Rexilius BG. *Chest drainage and suction.* Philadelphia: FA Davis; 1977.
Von Hippel A. *Chest tubes and chest bottles.* Springfield, IL: Charles C Thomas; 1970.

These two texts, the first by a registered nurse and the second by a surgeon, are excellent short volumes
that cover in greater detail the principles that have been condensed in this chapter. Both are recommended highly.

18

Management of Acute Pulmonary Disease

RESPIRATORY FAILURE

The purpose of the respiratory system is to oxygenate the blood and to remove carbon dioxide. Respiratory failure exists when oxygenation and/or carbon dioxide removal are inadequate. **Respiratory failure is defined as present when pO_2 is less than 60 mm Hg or pCO_2 is greater than 50 mm Hg.** These criteria identify presence of life-threatening respiratory dysfunction. Oxygenation may fail alone (hypoxia), CO_2 removal may fail alone (hypercapnia), or both respiratory functions may fail together (hypoxia and hypercapnia). Further deterioration in pO_2 or pCO_2 beyond these failure criteria may lead to cardiac and/or cerebral dysfunction and death on that basis. Also, once respiratory failure begins, rapid progression of abnormalities in pO_2 and pCO_2 may be seen, with consequent cardiopulmonary arrest. In fact, any hypercarbia significantly outside of the normal CO_2 range (up to pCO_2 46 mm Hg) should arouse concern. (Of course, many patients with chronic lung disease live long-term at levels of pO_2 and pCO_2 beyond the preceding criteria; these criteria for ventilatory failure apply to acute respiratory decompensation in patients without preexisting hypoxia or hypercarbia.)

Dyspnea and tachypnea are the usual clinical signs that signal respiratory failure and lead to the arterial blood gas determinations that confirm the diagnosis. Cyanosis may also be clinically apparent. Cardiac abnormalities (arrhythmia, hypertension) and neurologic abnormalities (confusion, obtundation, restlessness) may also signal respiratory failure and warrant ABG determination.

Rate and depth of respiration are important in the evaluation of hypercarbia. Slow, shallow respiration, as seen during sleep or from sedation by pain medications, implies that CO_2 retention may well be simply on the basis of suppression of respiratory drive, a transient and usually nonthreatening condition. Hypercarbia in face of

225

tachypnea and dyspnea has a much more ominous significance: This implies that CO_2 removal is failing despite maximal respiratory effort. Mild to moderate hypercarbia may also be seen as a compensation for metabolic alkalosis, in which case it is a normal phenomenon and not an expression of respiratory failure. (See "Acid-Base Nomogram" in Chapter 21.) This situation is seen most commonly in the ICU after very aggressive diuresis, with induction of the so-called hypokalemic, hypochloremic alkalosis of volume contraction.

Common causes of acute hypoxic respiratory failure in the ICU include atelectasis, pneumonia, pneumothorax, pulmonary edema, and pulmonary embolism. Common causes of acute hypercarbic respiratory failure include excess sedation, bronchospasm, atelectasis, pleural effusion, retained secretions, and respiratory muscle fatigue. In general, hypoxia implies perfused but underventilated alveoli, and hypercarbia implies ventilated but underperfused alveoli. (See Chapter 1.)

Treatment of respiratory failure is, of course, directed toward the underlying cause, which is determined in large part on the basis of physical examination and CXR. This treatment may include diuresis for pulmonary edema, broncholitics for bronchospasm, pulmonary toilet for retained secretions or atelectasis, and specific mechanical treatment for pneumothorax or effusion. Oxygen supplementation is, of course, indicated. **If immediate improvement is not seen with these measures, respiratory support by intubation and mechanical ventilation should be effected promptly—before a vicious cycle of deterioration ensues.** (The management of mechanical ventilation is reviewed in Chapter 1.) Intubation and mechanical ventilation are not infrequently required in the postoperative cardiac surgical patient, who may have atelectasis, effusion, an element of pulmonary edema, and muscle weakness. **The house officer should, when more experienced help is not available, always err on the side of early preemptive intubation for incipient respiratory failure.** Failure to do so, especially in the postinfarct or postoperative surgical patient, may result in cardiac arrest, from which recovery may be difficult. The period of mechanical ventilation, once instituted, allows time for correction of the underlying precipitating abnormalities.

ACUTE BRONCHOSPASM

Acute bronchospasm is commonly seen in ICU patients. After cardiac surgery, fluid overload and irritation of the airways related to intubation and retained secretions make patients vulnerable to bronchospasm. After acute myocardial infarction, a component of pulmonary edema may contribute to bronchospasm. Recognition of the bronchospastic attack is based on auscultation, usually occasioned by a call to the house officer to report that the patient is dyspneic. **During an attack of acute bronchospasm, significant hypoxia and/or significant hypercarbia on assessment of ABG's indicate a serious situation with potential for rapid deterioration.** Immediate treatment is required.

General modalities for treatment of acute bronchospasm in the ICU patient include the following:

1. **Oxygen administration**. Oxygen administration not only improves oxygen saturation, but also corrects the hyperventilation occasioned by acute bronchospasm, leading to less dyspnea and less work of breathing.
2. **Diuresis**. Especially after acute myocardial infarction or cardiac surgery, fluid overload with pulmonary edema causes airway edema, which narrows the small bronchi and may cause or exacerbate airway obstruction and bronchospasm. Lasix (40 mg IV) is almost always appropriate. When the emergency is corrected, attention to maintaining a net negative fluid balance over the next few days is important as well.
3. **Steroids**. We have found IV steroid administration to be extremely beneficial, especially for the bronchospasm frequently seen following extubation after cardiac surgery. Airway inflammation is improved promptly. We use hydrocortisone (100 mg IV q 8 h × 48 h). Even after cardiac surgery, a brief course of steroids does not lead to infectious complications. We find that by the end of the 48-h treatment period, the irritation of the airways and the clearance of secretions have improved markedly. We have found steroid treatment to be much better tolerated than theophylline administration in cardiac patients with bronchospasm.
4. **Inhaled bronchodilators**. The respiratory therapist will be able to offer a variety of inhalation treatments (including isoproterenol, metaproterenol, albuterol, and combinations of drugs), which will deliver bronchodilators topically into the airways to augment treatment of acute bronchospasm. Intravenous epinephrine or isoproterenol may also be useful (See Chapter 7).
5. **β-agonists**. β-agonists relax the bronchial smooth muscle. We have found terbutaline (0.25–0.5 mg sc q 4 h) a well-tolerated adjunct for relief of bronchospasm. We have not seen undue tachycardia or supraventricular or ventricular ectopy following treatment, and we actually prefer β-agonists to theophylline treatment in the post-MI or postoperative cardiac surgical patient.
6. **Theophylline**. We use IV aminophylline only as a last resort in post-MI and postoperative cardiac surgical patients, because in these settings supraventricular and ventricular ectopy is commonly induced by such treatment. We find that atrial fibrillation is almost invariably seen shortly after initiation of aminophylline treatment in the postoperative cardiac surgical patient. Moreover, the actual effectiveness of aminophylline as a bronchodilator has come into question (1). When we do use aminophylline, we err on the low side of recommended doses (5 mg/kg load over 20 min and 0.5 mg/kg/h maintenance), aiming for levels toward the low end of the therapeutic range (which is 10–20 mg/cc). Oral administration is better tolerated after acute MI or cardiac surgery, and despite our posture of avoiding IV aminophylline, we do at times treat even postinfarction and postoperative patients with oral theophylline (Theodur 200–300 mg p.o. q 12 h).
7. **Mechanical ventilation**. Because acute bronchospasm can deteriorate quickly, leading to life-threatening hypoxia and/or hypercarbia and cardiopulmonary ar-

rest, the house officer should maintain a low threshold for intubation and positive pressure ventilation in the setting of acute bronchospasm. Mechanical ventilation restores gas exchange immediately, providing time for institution of the other therapeutic modalities in a safe and timely fashion.

MASSIVE HEMOPTYSIS

Massive hemoptysis is defined as the expectoration of 600 cc or more of blood within a 24-h period. Such severe hemoptysis constitutes an emergency of the first order. Tuberculosis (with tuberculous cavity or penetrating hilar lymph node), chronic infection (bronchiectasis, lung abscess), and neoplasm are common causes of massive hemoptysis. **Death in hemoptysis occurs usually not from exsanguination, but from asphyxiation**, a principle that has important therapeutic correlates.

General supportive measures include the following: Hemostatic competence must be assured. All anticoagulant mediations must be discontinued. Aspirin-containing medications can be important culprits. Serious coagulation deficits can be corrected with fresh frozen plasma or platelets. The patient is positioned upright if neurologically intact or with the bleeding side down (decubitus position) if neurologically impaired, to prevent spilling of blood into the nonbleeding lung. Cough suppression with codeine is effected, to minimize mechanical disturbance of the bleeding lesion and local clot. Blood transfusion may be indicated if the hematocrit is low.

It is important to localize the site of bleeding. An alert patient often "senses" that the bleeding is coming from the right or the left side. The chest x-ray may be very helpful; the underlying lesion responsible for the hemoptysis (tumor, cavity) may be visible, or the "ground glass" appearance of aspirated blood in the parenchyma may localize the bleeding site. It is important to recognize that information from the x-ray may not be definitive; specifically, an endobronchial lesion different from the one apparent by chest x-ray may be the culprit, or aspirated blood may have drained to and opacified a lobe different from the one causing the bleeding.

Immediate bronchoscopic examination during the acute bleeding episode is key, as definitive localization of the bleeding site may be possible. We prefer rigid bronchoscopy because of the superior ability to clear endobronchial blood and clot in order to visualize the actual point of origin. Flexible bronchoscopy may suffice if rigid bronchoscopy is not available. Bronchoscopy of any type after the bleeding has ceased is often not definitive.

Because massive hemoptysis is life-threatening and tends to recur even after a specific episode has terminated, surgical treatment (usually by lobectomy) is the treatment of choice. Application of surgical treatment, however, presupposes that (1) the bleeding site has been identified definitively and (2) the patient is a suitable candidate for thoracic surgery. Often these conditions are not met. The site of bleeding may not be entirely clear. The patient often has significant underlying lung disease, and the acute hemoptysis may make precise assessment of pulmonary function inaccurate or unsafe. In the case of definitive localization of the site of hemoptysis and satisfactory general candidacy for operation, lobectomy constitutes definitive treatment.

Two general options are available for patients not deemed suitable candidates for operation: bronchial occlusion and bronchial artery embolization. Bronchial occlusion can be effected either by inflation of a balloon catheter in the mainstem bronchus of the bleeding lung or by intubation with a double-lumen tube (which allows ventilatory separation of the two lungs). Bronchial occlusion accomplishes two goals: It prevents aspiration of blood into the "good" lung, and it produces tamponade of the bleeding bronchus by trapping shed blood in the ipsilateral tree. At times, with bronchial occlusion, the whole lung on the affected side opacifies fully with shed blood. This almost always terminates the bleeding. Adequate oxygenation and ventilation are carried out using the "good" lung only. After 48–72 h, the bronchial blocker or double lumen tube is removed, allowing resumption of ventilation of the "bad" lung. The infiltrates usually clear in days to weeks, often without further hemoptysis.

Because massive hemoptysis usually originates pathologically from the high-pressure bronchial (not the low-pressure pulmonary) arteries, angiographic localization and bronchial artery embolization are feasible. This technique is fairly effective (2). The complication of paraplegia from inadvertent occlusion of the spinal artery, which may arise from the bronchial artery, can be devastating.

PULMONARY EMBOLISM

Pulmonary embolism is an extremely common cause of death in hospitalized patients, being seen in up to one of every four patients undergoing autopsy. Prevention is key. Although many adjuncts have been used—including subcutaneous heparin, Dextran, pneumatic calf compression, and antiembolism stockings—early and aggressive ambulation following myocardial infarction or cardiac surgery is essential for the prevention of pulmonary embolism.

An important principle is that **the hemodynamic disturbance from pulmonary embolism is caused not only by the occlusion of pulmonary artery radicles by the embolus itself, but also by the release of vasoactive amines into the pulmonary circulation, with consequent pulmonary artery vasoconstriction.** The vasoactive amines are released from the platelets involved in the continued thrombus deposition and destruction in, on, and around the main embolism. It is this vasoconstriction that raises pulmonary vascular resistance and pulmonary artery pressures, causing right heart strain, with elevation of central venous pressure and hemodynamic embarrassment up to and including cardiogenic shock. (The house officer should keep in mind that in standard pneumonectomy, one-half of the pulmonary vascular bed is acutely interrupted, usually without adverse hemodynamic sequelae. This observation emphasizes the pathologic importance of the vasoactive amine-induced pulmonary vasoconstriction that arises from pulmonary embolism but not from surgical pneumonectomy.)

Recognition of pulmonary embolism rests on maintaining a high index of suspicion. Cough, dyspnea, hypoxia, and pleuritic chest pain are well-known symptoms. These phenomena are seen even in the absence of pulmonary embolism in many postoperative cardiac surgical patients. If the symptoms seem at all out of the ordinary, we maintain a low threshold for diagnostic intervention.

Pulmonary embolism is extremely unlikely if the arterial pO_2 is not depressed. Some degree of hyperventilation usually accompanies the hypoxia of pulmonary embolism, leading to an arterial blood gas pattern of hypoxemia and hypocarbia (hyperventilation) in pulmonary embolism. This pattern is not, however, specific enough to rule in a pulmonary embolus.

Ventilation-perfusion lung scanning has proven a reasonable initial diagnostic test, which is less invasive than the gold standard of pulmonary arteriography. Magnetic resonance imaging (MRI) may prove an even more noninvasive alternative to pulmonary arteriography for detection of pulmonary embolism (3). Also, the cardiac ECHO, readily available at the bedside in coronary and postcardiac surgical ICUs, may detect thrombi still residing in right-sided cardiac chambers or in the main pulmonary arteries. The ECHO can supply other information relative to the diagnosis of pulmonary embolism, such as estimates of pulmonary artery pressure and of right ventricular strain. ECHO can also provide useful information about alternative diagnostic entities besides embolism in the acutely deteriorating patient, such as myocardial infarction, left ventricular dysfunction, aortic dissection, and pericardial effusion with tamponade. **Cardiac ECHO promises to play a larger role in the future in suspected pulmonary embolism** (4).

In the ICU setting, the question often arises whether an acute episode of hypotension or drop in cardiac output may be caused by pulmonary embolism. The Swan-Ganz catheter is very helpful in this regard. **It is very unlikely that hypotension is caused by acute pulmonary embolism if the central venous pressure and pulmonary artery systolic pressure are not acutely and markedly elevated.** Elevation of pulmonary artery pressure to the range of 50–60 mm Hg systolic and 30–40 mm Hg mean may be seen in acute massive pulmonary embolism. This helpful observation allows the house officer to focus his or her attention on other etiologies for hypotension without wasting precious time in the investigation for pulmonary embolism. Remember, however, that **the normal right ventricle cannot generate pressures higher than 60 mm Hg systolic with acute pulmonary embolism**; right heart failure ensues before pressure rises above this range with acute phenomena. This is in contradistinction to states of chronic pulmonary hypertension, where the hypertrophied right ventricle can generate systemic or even suprasystemic pressures.

The vast majority of patients with pulmonary embolism are adequately treated with intravenous heparin. Hemodynamics improve quickly, as the heparin terminates the cycle of clot formation and release of vasoactive amines. A loading dose of 5,000–10,000 U of heparin is used, followed by a continuous infusion of 800–1,200 U/h to maintain a PTT about one and a half to two times control. Coumadin is added orally after several days, and heparin is discontinued when, about 7–10 days postembolism, the PTT is therapeutic (one and a half to two times control).

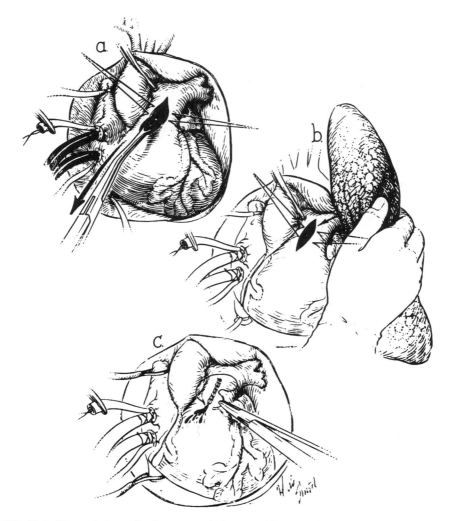

FIG. 18.1. The technique of pulmonary embolectomy. The procedure is most commonly performed on cardiopulmonary bypass, although on occasion when the heart-lung machine is not available, the original, nonbypass Trendelenburg procedure is performed. A longitudinal incision is made in the proximal pulmonary artery and clot is removed both directly and by compression of the lung.

In patients with severe hemodynamic compromise, thrombolytic therapy (urokinase, streptokinase, or rTPA) may be considered. These agents, which actually lyse fresh clots, lead to quicker hemodynamic improvement (5). In postoperative cardiac patients, however, thrombolytic therapy is usually contraindicated because of risk of bleeding from fresh operative sites and suture lines.

FIG. 18.2. Pulmonary arteriogram in a case of massive pulmonary embolism requiring operative pulmonary embolectomy on cardiopulmonary bypass because of refractory hypoxia and shock. The patient did well, with immediate correction of hypoxia and hemodynamic embarrassment.

In patients who manifest refractory hemodynamic embarrassment or hypoxia despite mechanical intubation and positive pressure ventilation, inotropic support, and anticoagulation with heparin and/or thrombolysis, emergency surgical performance of pulmonary embolectomy may be indicated. Although the operative risk is high, reflecting the desperate condition of the patients, hemodynamics may be restored immediately in selected patients and salvage effected. Although originally performed by Trendelenburg without the heart-lung machine, pulmonary embolectomy is currently performed on cardiopulmonary bypass. (See Figs. 18.1 and 18.2.)

REFERENCES

1. Littenberg B. Aminophylline treatment in severe, acute asthma: a meta-analysis. *JAMA* 1988;259:1678–1684.
2. Magilligan DJ, Jr, Ravipoti S, Zayat P, Shetty PC, Bower G, Kvale P. Massive hemoptysis: control by transcatheter bronchial embolization. *Ann Thorac Surg* 1981;32:392–400.
3. White RD, Winkler ML, Higgins CB. MR imaging of pulmonary arterial hypertension and pulmonary emboli. *American Journal of Roentgenology* 1987;149:15–21.

4. Torbicki A, Tramarin R, Morpurgo M. Role of echo/doppler in the diagnosis of pulmonary embolism. *Clin Cardiol* 1992;15:805–810.
5. Cuccia C, Campana M, Frajnzoni P, Faggiano P, Volterrani M, Musmeci G, Visioli O. Effectiveness of intravenous rTPA in the treatment of massive pulmonary embolism and right heart thromboembolism. *Am Heart J* 1993;126:468–472.

SUGGESTED FURTHER READING

Hyers TM, ed. Pulmonary embolism and hypertension. *Clin Chest Med* 1984;5:383–554.

An entire text devoted to the subject of pulmonary embolism—authoritative, complete, and interesting to read.

Knott-Craig, CJ, Oostuizen JG, Rossouw G, Joubert JR, Barnard PM. Management and prognosis of massive hemoptysis: recent experience with 120 patients. *J Thorac Cardiovasc Surg* 1993;105:394–397.

An up-to-date review in a large number of patients, which looks not only at results in terms of survival to hospital discharge, but at subsequent survival as well.

19 Problems Following Noncardiac Thoracic Surgery

Five major categories of problems can occur acutely following chest surgery, including thoracotomy, lung biopsy, lobectomy, and pneumonectomy:

Bleeding
Arrhythmias
Space problems
Volume loss in remaining lung tissue
Congestive heart failure

Each of these categories requires the understanding and awareness of the house officer.

BLEEDING

Major bleeding can follow lobectomy or pneumonectomy. Not only may a ligature come off a pulmonary artery or vein, but the fragile pulmonary artery may tear at the site of an intact ligature (from continued beat-by-beat trauma). Bleeding from a major vessel will usually result in rapid compromise of vital signs. A dramatic volume of bleeding through the chest tubes will usually be evident.

Urgent reoperation may be necessary. Rarely, reoperation in the ICU may be necessary. Such interventions may on occasion be life-saving. **Almost all sites of bleeding can be controlled by manual compression** until expert surgical assistance and proper lighting and equipment are available. Blind application of traumatic nonvascular clamps must be avoided.

Aside from bleeding from major vessels, considerable oozing may occur from denuded parenchymal surfaces, especially when incomplete fissures are opened bluntly or when adherent, inflamed pleural surfaces are separated. The surgeon will achieve meticulous hemostasis in the operating room. Still, several hundred milliliters of bleeding per hour may occasionally be seen early after thoracic surgery. The house officer should alert senior personnel of such bleeding but must not panic. As parenchymal surfaces appose to the parietal pleura, bleeding from raw tissues will stop. Assuring full expansion of the lung is important for this reason.

As will be discussed later, pneumonectomy is often performed without indwelling chest tubes. Bleeding is more common after pneumonectomy, because there is no parenchymal surface to appose onto the pleura. Without a chest tube in place, significant bleeding may not be obvious. If deterioration of vital signs or falling hematocrit suggest bleeding, a chest x-ray (CXR) will allow assessment of fluid volume on the side of pneumonectomy. Normally after pneumonectomy, the space fills with fluid over days to weeks (Fig. 19.1). **A rapid rise in fluid level in the pneumonectomy space in the first hours postoperatively suggests bleeding.**

ARRHYTHMIAS

The same supraventricular arrhythmias that follow cardiac surgery may follow thoracic surgery. Their management is detailed in Chapter 2.

Usually the thoracic surgical patient has a healthier heart than the cardiac surgical patient. The former usually tolerates supraventricular tachycardia better, allowing the house officer a longer safety margin in treatment.

Traditionally, many surgeons prophylactically digitalize the elderly patient who undergoes lobectomy or pneumonectomy. Many surgeons use a cutoff of 60 or 65 years of age. Much debate has been carried out over the years regarding the benefits and risks of prophylactic digitalization. The main benefit is that the digitalized patient who goes into atrial fibrillation does so at a controlled rate. The risk is that, especially with potassium fluxes, digitalis toxicity may be seen. This issue was more germane in earlier years, when digitalis was the only available agent. Now that intravenous β-blockers and calcium antagonists are available, immediate control of rate when atrial fibrillation occurs is attained more easily than before; this affords time for "after-the-fact" digitalization.

SPACE PROBLEMS

After lobectomy, a variety of compensatory mechanisms allow the space previously occupied by the excised lobe to be filled: The remaining lobe overexpands; the mediastinum moves to the operated side; the diaphragm moves up; the ribs move closer together. Most often, these mechanisms, combined with proper chest tube placement, result in the remaining lobe's completely filling the pleural cavity. **Occasionally, after lobectomy the pleural cavity may not be filled entirely.** The house officer must follow postoperative CXRs closely and call any remaining major space (pneumothorax) to the attention of senior staff. A number of manipulations of the drainage systems are available to overcome such a problem. These are carried out at the judgment and discretion of the surgeon.

Another reason incomplete expansion is important regards the postoperative air leak. **Air leak is normal after pulmonary surgery.** Parenchymal areas of adhesion and incomplete fissures will leak air of necessity. (The bronchial stump, of course, must be closed totally securely.) These parenchymal leaks will usually seal within hours of complete apposition of the lung to the chest wall. If an air space remains, some parenchyma may not adhere to the visceral pleura and may continue to leak for days.

Special consideration must be paid to postpneumonectomy space problems. After pneumonectomy, the same mechanisms (mediastinal shift, diaphragmatic elevation, and narrowing of intercostal spaces) serve to minimize the empty space in the operated thorax. **The compensatory mechanisms cannot, however, totally obliterate the postpneumonectomy space, as no lung remains on the operated side.** Over days to weeks, that space will fill with fluid, which will eventually form an organized coagulum.

On the first night after thoracic surgery, postpneumonectomy space problems may cause major hemodynamic abnormality (1–5), as a result of shifts in mediastinal position. Some surgeons believe that the mediastinum shifts toward the unoperated side most commonly, because fluid is secreted more rapidly than air is absorbed from the postpneumonectomy space. Other surgeons believe that the mediastinum shifts most commonly toward the operated side, because fluid secretion lags behind air absorption. Other factors may be relevant. When the patient is turned from the lateral decubitus position to the supine position at the completion of the resection, the diaphragm may be pushed up by intra-abdominal contents, with increase in pressure on the operated side and displacement of the mediastinum toward the unoperated side. On the other hand, at times air may be pushed through the chest wall closure into the soft tissues or the atmosphere, resulting in net negative pressure in the postpneumonectomy space and shift of the mediastinum to the operated side. It is best for the house officer to conclude that, **in particular cases, following pneumonectomy, significant mediastinal shift may occur toward either the operated or the unoperated side**.

Shift in either direction may cause major hemodynamic upset. Significant shift toward the operated side may occlude the great veins and impair cardiac filling. Shift toward the unoperated side may impair function of the sole remaining lung. Mediastinal shift has also been implicated as a cause of arrhythmias following pneumonectomy.

When hemodynamic instability occurs following pneumonectomy, mediastinal position must be assessed immediately. In fact, the house officer should monitor mediastinal position regularly to *prevent* excess deviation. Feeling for deviation of the trachea and percussing for location of the left ventricular apex may give some valuable clinical information regarding mediastinal displacement. Above all other tests, however, **it is the CXR that allows precise assessment of mediastinal position.** The CXR must be taken squarely anteroposterior or posteroanterior; minor ro-

FIG. 19.1. Chest x-rays showing progressive filling of the postpneumonectomy space by fluid with time. **A:** Preoperative. Note lesion in the left mid-lung field. **B:** Postoperative, with tubes in place emptying pleural space.

C

D

FIG. 19.1. *(continued)* **C:** Five days postoperatively. **D:** Ten days postoperatively. Note rising fluid level in **C** and **D**. The pleural space will eventually fill entirely with fluid.

tation of the x-ray may cause misleading contours. Usually, the mediastinal shifts are obvious if they are the cause of hemodynamic instability. In contralateral shift, the remaining lung will be seen to be severely compressed. In ipsilateral shift, the heart shadow may lie against the chest wall.

Mediastinal shift must be corrected when it is severe in extent or when it causes hemodynamic embarrassment. Most surgeons close the chest following pneumonectomy without an indwelling chest tube. Shift toward the unoperated side (by excess positive pressure in the pneumonectomy space) is corrected by aspirating air by needle and syringe until mediastinal position normalizes. Shift toward the operated side (by excess negative pressure in the pneumonectomy space) is corrected by injecting air by needle and syringe until mediastinal position normalizes. Aspirations or injections must be done with strict aseptic technique, as the empty pneumonectomy space infects easily. The house officer must discuss all manipulations with senior staff experienced in postpneumonectomy space problems.

Some surgeons do leave a tube to simple water seal following pneumonectomy. (This tube must *never* be placed to suction; this would cause high negative pressure and fatal ipsilateral shift.) When this system is used, the tube is withdrawn from water seal once hourly to allow equilibration with atmospheric pressure. The level of water in the straw serves as a water manometer, allowing continuous assessment of intrapleural pressure. (See Chapter 17.) The ideal postpneumonectomy pressure is mildly negative (approximately 2–6 cm H_2O). (If a particular surgeon uses this chest tube system following pneumonectomy, the house officer must review in detail the surgeon's instructions for manipulations.) In this system, the tube is removed the morning after surgery.

A relatively new chest drainage system (a special postpneumonectomy Pleurevac from Deknatel, Inc.) automatically controls pressure in the postpneumonectomy space; by virtue of two water-seal chambers, this special device continually allows air to enter or exit the space to keep pressure within selected parameters. This system eliminates the need for the house officer to "lift the straw hourly from the water reservoir." This is an ingenious system that essentially eliminates postpneumonectomy hemodynamic instability related to mediastinal shift. This device takes over the house officer's responsibility reliably. Not all surgeons employ this device, however.

Hemodynamic compromise from mediastinal shift is unlikely after the immediate postoperative night. By the following morning, the circulatory system has usually adapted to minor shifts and the mediastinum begins to fix its position by edema and fibrosis. CXR position is still monitored daily, but adjustments rarely need be made.

VOLUME LOSS

It is very common on the first, second, or third postoperative days to see significant or even total atelectasis in the lung tissue remaining after lobectomy. Many factors encourage this atelectasis. Even an optimal resection may narrow, by edema, the remaining bronchial tree. Viscid secretions are exacerbated by premedication and anesthesia and may plug bronchi. Postoperative pain discourages deep breathing. The house officer must carefully assess and follow aeration of the remaining lobes. If aeration appears to be diminishing, pulmonary toilet must be intensified. Analgesics must be given to allow deep breathing and coughing. Incentive spirometer exercises must be emphasized. Endotracheal suctioning may be necessary.

If total atelectasis develops and does not respond overnight to intensive bronchopulmonary toilet measures, bronchoscopy should be carried out. Our preference is for rigid bronchoscopy, which permits excellent suctioning of secretions and plugs. Many use flexible bronchoscopy. When total atelectasis occurs, of course, the house officer must follow arterial blood gases closely, as considerable shunting and hypoxia can occur. Once chest tubes are out and the patient is up and about, full expansion usually is maintained by normal respiratory excursion.

After pneumonectomy, of course, no lobe remains on the operated side. It is not uncommon, however, to see infiltrates on the side of the nonoperated, dependent lung. The house officer should expect to see these CXR changes, which reflect secretions draining into the dependent lung during the procedure. These infiltrates usually clear overnight.

CONGESTIVE HEART FAILURE

Pulmonary resection decreases the vascular bed through which the right heart can pump; in effect, pulmonary vascular resistance is raised, raising right ventricular afterload and pulmonary artery pressures. This is especially significant after pneumonectomy, where half the pulmonary vascular bed is removed. Though a normal healthy lung compensates for occlusion of a single pulmonary artery, this often is not the case in operated patients, whose remaining lung may be afflicted with preexisting pulmonary disease (1).

Additionally, the lung remaining after pneumonectomy is liable to be flooded easily (2,6). It is best to run these patients "dry." Pneumonectomy carries a considerable mortality. Right heart failure is one important factor. Right heart function is best followed by keeping track of central venous pressure. In fact, the Swan-Ganz catheter is almost contraindicated. It cannot safely be placed preoperatively, because it may go into the portion of the lung to be resected (unless fluoroscopic control is utilized). Placing the Swan-Ganz catheter postoperatively may carry the danger of disruption of the pulmonary artery stump by the advancing catheter. In any case, left heart function is usually normal; function of the right heart is well assessed by a simple central venous pressure catheter.

PULMONARY EMBOLISM

One important recent paper (7) has focused specifically on thromboembolism following pulmonary resection. With careful screening by pre- and postoperative venous duplex and ventilation-perfusion scanning, it was found that 25% of patients had deep vein thrombosis and/or pulmonary embolism following pulmonary resection. Thromboembolic disease was more common in patients with bronchogenic carcinoma (compared to other causes for resection), larger tumors (compared to small tumors), and larger resections (pneumonectomy or lobectomy compared to segmentectomy and wedge resection). The house officer should keep pulmonary embolism in mind in the postthoracotomy patient, especially since the postthoracotomy state may obscure the common manifestations of pulmonary embolism (pain, dyspnea, effusion, hypoxia).

ADDITIONAL PROBLEMS

Two other conditions can cause major instability early after thoracic procedures. These will be covered briefly, for they are rare.

Lobar Torsion

Torsion of a remaining lobe may occur. This results from surgical division of normal stabilizing attachments (including incomplete fissures, pulmonary ligaments, and mediastinal pleural attachments). The surgeon will often fix the remaining lobe with sutures to prevent torsion. When torsion does occur, severe toxicity results; the lobe will progress to gangrene if the condition is not recognized. A hazy appearance of the lobe on CXR (2) may suggest torsion. Bronchoscopy may confirm the diagnosis, as a twisted lobar bronchus can be seen (8). Urgent reexploration and resection of the affected lobe must be carried out immediately.

Cardiac Herniation

When the pericardium has been opened for intrapericardial pneumonectomy, herniation of the heart may occur through the defect. This unusual complication is lethal unless immediate operation and reduction are carried out. CXR may confirm the diagnosis, but there may not be sufficient time to obtain and develop the film. The key is prevention at the time of surgery by closing even small pericardial defects. An awareness of this disorder and an index of suspicion for it on the part of the house officer may be life-saving.

One additional comment should be made concerning mechanical ventilation of the patient after pulmonary resection. Many chest surgeons, the authors included, feel it is important to extubate the patient as soon as possible after thoracic surgery, preferably on the operating table before transfer. Prolonged ventilation may be deleterious in a number of ways. Positive pressure puts extra strain on the bronchial stump and encourages parenchymal air leaks. Prolonged intubation stimulates tracheobronchial secretions and interferes with mucosal defense mechanisms of the bronchial tree. With careful selection of patients preoperatively, on-the-table extubation will be possible in the vast majority of cases.

REFERENCES

1. Young W, Perryman, R. Complications of pneumonectomy. In: Cordell A, Ellison R, eds. *Complications of intrathoracic surgery*. Boston: Little, Brown 1979:257–266.
2. Kirsh M, Rotman H, Behrendt D, et al. Complications of pulmonary resection. *Ann Thorac Surg* 1975;20:216–236.
3. Maier H. Pneumonectomy: methods of improving morbidity and mortality rates. *Surg Clin North Am* 1962;42:1527–1536.
4. Von Hippel A. *A manual of thoracic surgery*. Springfield, IL: Charles C Thomas, 1978.
5. Langston, H, Barker, W. The adult thoracic surgical patient. In: Neville W, ed. *Intensive care of the surgical cardiopulmonary patient*. Chicago: Year Book; 1983:235–261.
6. Gibbon J, Gibbon M, Kraul, C. Experimental pulmonary edema following lobectomy and blood transfusion. *J Thorac Surg* 1942;12:60.
7. Ziomek S, Read RC, Tobler HG, et al. Thromboembolism in patients undergoing thoracotomy. *Ann Thorac Surg* 1993;56:223–227.
8. Brooks J. Complications following pulmonary lobectomy. In: Cordell A, Ellison R, eds. *Complications of intrathoracic surgery*. Boston: Little, Brown; 1979;235–256.

SUGGESTED FURTHER READING

Kirsh M, Rotman H, Behrendt D, et al. Complications of pulmonary resection. *Ann Thorac Surg* 1975;20:216–236.

A clearly written and inclusive review with illustrative x-rays.

20 Aortic Emergencies

Thoracic aortic emergencies include acute **aortic transection, rupture of thoracic aortic aneurysm,** and **acute aortic dissection.** These are distinct entities often confused by house officers and practitioners alike. Much of this confusion stems from unfortunate terminology. Nonetheless, these conditions are among the most dangerous and challenging that the house officer faces in the coronary or surgical intensive care units. Before addressing specifically the role of the junior house officer in the management of aortic emergencies, certain general matters of orientation will be clarified.

TYPES OF AORTIC PATHOLOGY

Acute aortic dissection should be distinguished clearly from acute transections of the thoracic aorta and from chronic "arteriosclerotic" aneurysms of the thoracic or abdominal aorta (Fig. 20.1).

Acute Aortic Transection

Acute transections of the thoracic aorta follow severe blunt trauma. The aortic wall is torn, often circumferentially, and at times transmurally. This condition is often immediately fatal because of exsanguination. Those who survive to reach the emergency center have the tear contained by the adventitia and pleural tissue overlying the aorta, preventing exsanguination. The aorta itself is intrinsically normal prior to the injury. The wall has normal strength. The layers of the wall do not split from each other for any significant distance—indeed, they cannot, because the basic consistency of the tissues is normal. This disorder is merely a tearing, not a dissection. It requires urgent repair through the left chest, which is often done without cardiopulmonary bypass. A

245

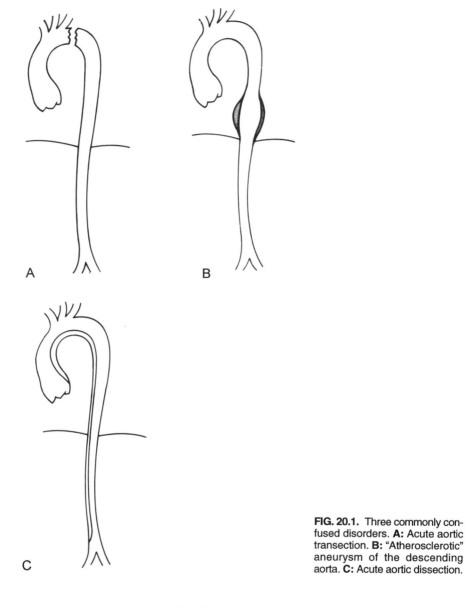

FIG. 20.1. Three commonly confused disorders. **A:** Acute aortic transection. **B:** "Atherosclerotic" aneurysm of the descending aorta. **C:** Acute aortic dissection.

short prosthetic graft is placed end to end to replace the aorta at the site of the tear (Fig. 20.2); occasionally, the native tissues may be approximated primarily.

A high index of suspicion for this disorder is essential. This message has been well promulgated, and most house officers are well aware they they should suspect this injury in any victim of high-speed deceleration injury, especially in face of medi-

FIG. 20.2. Operative procedure for acute aortic transection. A short Dacron graft is inserted at the site of transection just beyond the subclavian artery. (Reprinted with permission from Ref. 12.)

astinal widening or loss of clarity of the aortic knob or the stripe of the descending aorta on x-ray examination. The diagnostic investigation for this suspected disorder is currently in flux, as discussed in Chapter 11, although aortography remains the gold standard.

The treatment in suspected cases, or in documented cases before operative intervention is performed, is **strict blood pressure control**. In patients young and healthy except for the traumatic event, we keep blood pressure at 80–90 mm Hg systolic. In case operative intervention needs to be delayed, β-blockers can be added to decrease the strength of cardiac contraction.

Chronic "Arteriosclerotic" Aneurysms

Chronic "arteriosclerotic" aneurysms of the thoracic and abdominal aorta result from weakening of the aortic wall and fusiform dilatation. The abdominal aorta distal to the renal arteries is most commonly affected. Rarely, the process may extend proximally to the level of the renal arteries. The thoracic aorta is less commonly involved than the abdominal aorta. When the thoracic aorta is involved, the aneurysm is usually in the descending aorta. Inside the fusiform dilatation, one finds organized, laminated thrombus. Although the aorta itself at the aneurysm is markedly abnormal, it has stretched concentrically, not dissected longitudinally. The layers of the aortic wall are normally adherent. Such dilatation of the aorta has long been considered to be of arteriosclerotic origin. This concept has recently been challenged, with an inherited metabolic predisposition coming to light (1,2). Nonetheless, dissection of one

FIG. 20.3. Operative procedure for "arteriosclerotic" aneurysm of the descending aorta. The aneurysm is opened and replaced by a long Dacron graft, which is then wrapped with the wall of the aneurysm. (Reproduced with permission from Ref. 13.)

layer of the aortic wall from another is not part of this process. These aneurysms can rupture; they do not commonly dissect. Surgery is carried out electively when these aneurysms reach a size at which rupture becomes a significant danger. Most surgeons operate when the diameter of the descending aorta reaches 6 or 8 cm or begins to change rapidly. A prosthetic graft is used to replace the diseased aorta, with or without cardiopulmonary bypass (Fig. 20.3). If the ascending aorta is involved by such an aneurysm cardiopulmonary bypass is required for the repair. When these aneurysms do rupture, bleeding may be contained by mediastinal pleural tissues or by the retroperitoneal tissues. When the emergency physician calls to report a "dissecting" abdominal aneurysm, he does not mean that at all, but rather an abdominal aneurysm that has ruptured but remains contained. The same applies for rupture of this condition in the thorax.

Acute Aortic Dissection

Acute aortic dissection refers to a specific condition in which the layers of the aorta are split from each other, with blood under pressure entering between the layers and

FIG. 20.4. Gross pathology specimen of a descending aorta involved by acute aortic dissection. The true lumen is below and to the left, and the false channel is above and to the right. (Reproduced with permission from Ref. 13.)

FIG. 20.5. Types I, II, and III aortic dissections.

propagating the split to various extents. This process begins with a tear through the intima and inner media at one specific site. Blood under pressure gains access within the media and forces its separation into layers (3). The split occurs within the tunica media. The intima and inner media are forced inward. The outer media and adventitia are forced outward (Fig. 20.4). This separation of layers is the "dissection." It is an acute process that occurs in a chronically degenerated aorta. At one instant the dissection is not present. At the next instant, the initial tear occurs and the dissection propagates. The degeneration of the aortic wall that allows this to occur is a chronic process. Long-standing hypertension is thought to be the most important predisposing factor. Connective tissue disorders (especially Marfan's syndrome) are other predisposing conditions. With each hypertensive beat, the aorta is battered. The media in particular is weakened. After years of weakening, the media degenerates to the point where the initial tear and the dissection can occur (3).

It is the use of the term *dissecting aneurysm of the aorta* that fosters confusion with chronic "arteriosclerotic" aneurysms. It is best not to think of acute aortic dissection as an aneurysm at all. Until the acute phenomenon occurs, the aorta is of normal caliber. After the split occurs, although the aorta usually has widened, it is the splitting of layers that has caused the widening that constitutes the crucial pathophysiologic event. It is best to term this acute phenomenon an "acute aortic dissection" rather than an "aneurysm" of any type.

There are three basic types of acute aortic dissections (Fig. 20.5). In types I and II, the initiating intimal tear occurs in the **ascending** aorta. In type I, the dissection propagates beyond the ascending aorta, often into the aorta arch, down the descending aorta, down the abdominal aorta, and into the iliacs. In type II, the dissection confines itself to the ascending aorta. In type III, the dissection begins in the **descending** aorta, beyond the left subclavian artery, and then propagates distally. The important point for the house officer is to be aware that **the initial tear in aortic dissection tends to occur in two very specific locations: about 4 cm above the aortic valve in ascending dissection, and just beyond the subclavian artery in descending dissection. Management guidelines are based strongly on the location—ascending or descending—of the initial tear.**

SEQUELAE OF AORTIC DISSECTION

Dissection can cause several general categories of harm to the patient (Fig. 20.6).

Rupture

The force of pulsatile blood may break through the outer medial-adventitial layer, causing rupture of the aorta into the pericardium or, more rarely, into the chest or abdomen. Exsanguination can occur rapidly if the rupture is free. Bleeding may be contained to some degree by the fibrous tissue investing the descending thoracic and abdominal aorta, as well as the pleural or peritoneal tissues.

Tamponade

The pericardium attaches to the aorta several centimeters above the aortic valve along the ascending aorta. The ascending aorta lies freely in the pericardial cavity, surrounded by a thin layer of epicardium. For this reason, a dissection involving the ascending aorta can rupture into the pericardium. This can cause tamponade of varying severity.

Branch Occlusion

Flow through any of the branches of the aortic arch, descending aorta, or abdominal aorta may be occluded by the dissection. This occurs because pressure in the false lumen compromises the true lumen (Fig. 20.7). Involvement of the innominate or carotid arteries can cause stroke. Involvement of the innominate or subclavian arteries can result in arm ischemia. Involvement of the thoracic intercostals can render the spinal cord ischemic, with resultant paraplegia. Involvement of mesenteric vessels can cause intestinal ischemia. Involvement of the renal arteries can cause renal failure and Goldblatt-type hypertension. Involvement of the iliac or femoral arteries can

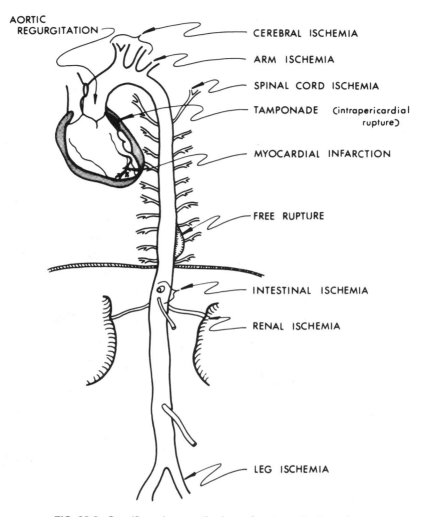

FIG. 20.6. Specific major complications of acute aortic dissection.

result in lower-extremity ischemia. Also, the coronary arteries themselves can become involved, resulting in myocardial ischemia or infarction.

Aortic Regurgitation

The dissection in the ascending aorta (in types I and II) can "unseat" the aortic valve from its annulus, resulting in acute aortic regurgitation. This disorder is usually very poorly tolerated. Severe congestive heart failure or cardiogenic shock often follow quickly.

FIG. 20.7. Schematic representation of the mechanism by which aortic dissection can "pinch off" an arterial branch of the aorta. **A:** The dissection process with branch vessel occlusion. **B:** Relief of occlusion by the "fenestration" procedure (see later).

SPECIFIC CARE

The role of the house officer in caring for patients with acute aortic dissection will be discussed under several headings: recognition, assessment, management decisions, preoperative care, operative management, and postoperative care.

Recognition

The burden of recognition usually falls on the medical house officer in the emergency department or the coronary care unit. The patient with an acute aortic dissection has pain in the chest and/or the thoracic back. He or she is usually triaged with patients who have angina or myocardial infarction. The excruciating nature of the pain and the association with pain in the back should arouse suspicion that dissection may be occurring. Absence of EKG changes of ischemia may lead to further suspicion that the process is not myocardial ischemia. Ischemic EKG changes, however,

FIG. 20.8. Presenting chest x-ray of a patient with acute aortic dissection. The type I dissection involved the ascending aorta, the aortic arch, and the descending aorta; widening of the contour of each of these aortic segments can be discerned.

do not necessarily rule out an acute aortic dissection, since coronary involvement can be a sequel of the dissection. A history of long-standing hypertension also should raise suspicion. The chest x-ray (CXR) is the key in differentiating patients with dissection from the many with ischemic pain. The shadows of the ascending aorta, the aortic knob, and the descending aorta will be widened and distorted when these segments are involved (Fig. 20.8). Also, the physical findings of injury according to the four patterns described earlier—rupture, tamponade, branch occlusion, and aortic regurgitation—can be quite specific, as in the case of loss of a peripheral pulse or development of a new diastolic murmur. **A patient in whom the suspicion of acute dissection exists should undergo urgent aortography or one of the other more modern alternative imaging modalities**. (See Chapter 11.)

The house officer should note that acute aortic dissection is **not** rare. **Acute dissection is, in fact, the most common acute catastrophe involving the human aorta**, occurring even more commonly than rupture of abdominal "atherosclerotic" aneurysms

(3–5). It is lack of recognition that accounts for the impression that this disorder is unusual.

Assessment

The house officer must assess the type of dissection: Is it ascending or descending? This can be usually done on the basis of symptoms, physical exam, and CXR. Ascending dissection presents with anterior chest pain while descending dissection presents with pain in the thoracic back. The house officer must ascertain as well which of the sequelae of dissection has occurred.

Intrathoracic rupture will cause a left hemothorax to appear on CXR. Intra-abdominal rupture will lead to peritoneal signs. Tamponade will present as described in Chapter 16. Occlusion of carotid or arm or leg arteries will be apparent from absent pulses and ischemia in the involved vascular distributions. Coronary occlusion will usually manifest on EKG. Renal occlusion will show as oliguria, anuria, or intractable hypertension. Intestinal ischemia is the most difficult to detect; peritoneal signs may not follow for many hours. If the patient is having any nausea or abdominal discomfort, or if there is abdominal distention, intestinal involvement is likely. Spinal cord ischemia shows as distal sensory/motor disturbance.

Aortic valve involvement will produce symptoms and signs of congestive heart failure or pulmonary edema. It is critical to listen for the murmur of aortic regurgitation.

On the basis of history, physical exam, and CXR, the house officer should be able to formulate a good assessment of the type of dissection and the extent of its complications. Angiography (and/or CT, ECHO, or MRI) will corroborate and amplify. This assessment will allow decisions regarding whether surgery is indicated and, when necessary, which surgical procedure should be performed.

Management Decisions

Though management of acute dissections remains controversial and complex, the general principles regarding surgical management used at our institution can be simplified as follows. (Practice at some institutions may differ; this simplified paradigm is intended to provide the house officer with some orientation for decision making in this complex disorder.)

Ascending dissections require urgent surgery, if for no other reason than because the risk of fatal intrapericardial rupture exists. The process of intrapericardial rupture has often begun before the patient's presentation to the hospital. Some time usually intervenes between the onset of intrapericardial bleeding and flagrant tamponade with complete failure of cardiac function. More often than not, for ascending dissections, other complications, especially occlusion of important branch vessels and unseating of the aortic valve, would require intervention even if intrapericardial rupture did not occur. For this reason, ascending dissections represent surgical lesions.

Descending dissections are generally treated medically (see later) unless specific complications necessitate surgical intervention (4,5). Some authorities disagree and consider these lesions surgical as well (6). Free rupture can usually be prevented by prompt and sustained blood pressure control. If vital branch vessels have been occluded by the dissection, however, surgery must be carried out. Barring unpreventable rupture or major vessel occlusion, descending dissections are medical lesions.

Preoperative Care

Specific preoperative care comprises two basic endeavors:

1. Blood pressure must be controlled.
2. Continued reassessment of extent of dissection and complications incurred must be carried out.

In patients being treated for dissection—either before surgery, after surgery, or in place of surgery—blood pressure must be strictly controlled. Blood pressure must be reduced to the minimum levels that will sustain life and adequate organ function. Usually, we like to see **systolic blood pressure of 100 mm Hg or less.** Higher pressures increase the likelihood that each heartbeat will rupture the thin adventitia or propagate the dissection further.

In the acute setting, continuous infusion of sodium nitroprusside (Nipride) or trimethaphan (Arfonad) is very effective in controlling blood pressure to any level desired. Particulars regarding use of continuous infusion agents are covered in Chapter 7. Nifedipine (10–20 mg) given sublingually can be very useful as an initial measure during transport or while the continuous infusions are being prepared.

Intravenous propranolol (Inderal) is given at intervals to help with blood pressure control. It is thought by some that, by impairing contractility and decreasing the rate of rise of systemic pressure with each heart beat, β-blockers may be specifically indicated in treating aortic dissection; presumably, the forcefulness of each heartbeat is diminished. Labetalol is a newer agent that is being used in dissection as an alternative to Inderal (7). In addition to being a β-blocker, this drug also produces peripheral vasodilation, which enhances blood pressure control. This medication can be given by continuous infusion; an initial bolus of 20 mg can be followed by an infusion of 2 mg/min. This drug has a long half-life (6–8 h). Continuous infusion should be discontinued when control of heart rate and blood pressure are achieved to avoid cumulative toxicity.

When transition to chronic oral therapy is made, we usually use an afterload-reducing agent (such as hydralazine or nifedipine; see Chapter 21) and a β-blocker (such as Inderal). Blood pressure limits are liberalized only slightly for chronic control.

The house officer must be aware, especially in the acute setting, that inducing low or normal blood pressure in these patients with chronic, severe hypertension may, while treating the dissection, impair specific organ function. If the patient has cerebral, coronary, or renal artery disease, the reduced pressure head may prove insufficient for perfusion of the respective vascular beds. If mental obtundation or oliguria develops, the intravenous infusion should be titrated down to ensure adequate cerebral and/or renal perfusion.

Operative Management

The house officer must have some basic understanding of the methods of surgical correction of these complex disorders in order to care for the patient preoperatively and postoperatively. Again, for purposes of clarity, operative procedures will be simplified in this discussion, so that the house officer may concentrate on developing a fundamental perspective.

Ascending dissections are treated by replacement of the ascending aorta (Fig. 20.9). The segment of aorta between the aortic valve and the aortic arch—the segment in which the intimal tear resides—is excised and replaced by a graft. This is done on cardiopulmonary bypass. Occasionally, for technical reasons, this operation must be done under deep hypothermia with circulatory arrest—a type of "suspended animation" in which the heart-lung machine is turned off for a period of time (8). Replacing this specific segment of aorta accomplishes several important goals. Future rupture into the pericardium is prevented. The intimal tear is removed, so that blood under pressure no longer enters the false lumen through that tear. This usually suffices to restore blood supply to branches occluded by the dissection. If blood supply is not restored to a particular branch system, further treatment (as for descending dissection, discussed later) may be required. The ascending aortic replacement (depicted in Fig. 20.9) does not eliminate the remainder of the dissected aorta; for this reason, lifelong blood pressure control is required afterward.

In ascending dissections, if the aortic valve has been unseated by the dissection, the valve is repaired or replaced at the time that the ascending aorta is replaced. This eliminates the acute aortic regurgitation that is often quickly fatal if not corrected.

For descending dissections, we have advocated what we call the *complication-specific approach* (9) (Fig. 20.10). In this approach, if no complications occur, descending dissection is treated medically. If complications do occur, operation is carried out, with the specific operation determined by the specific complication. Frank rupture is treated by replacement of the descending aorta by a Dacron graft. Impending rupture (manifested by rapid enlargement) is treated by an ingenious operation developed by Professor Alain Carpentier of France (10). In this operation, an extra-anatomic pathway is created to replace the descending aorta; the descending aorta itself is permanently occluded by a clamp, allowing gradual thrombosis of the entire descending thoracic aorta (Fig. 20.11). If the complication is branch occlusion and organ ischemia (most commonly, occlusion of an iliac artery with leg ischemia), the "fenestration" procedure is performed, accomplishing decompression of the false lumen and restoring blood flow to the affected organ (11) (Fig. 20.12). This procedure is quite effec-

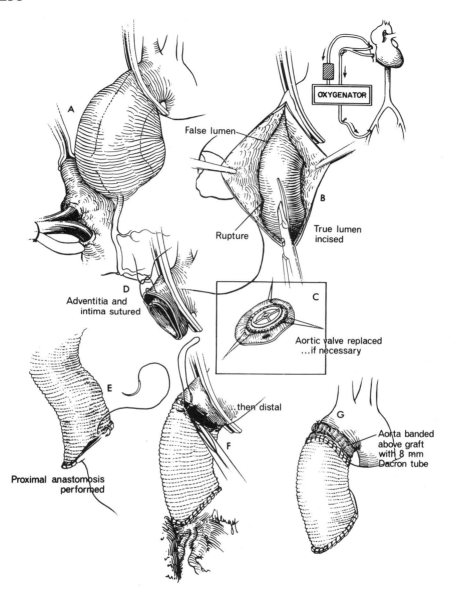

FIG. 20.9. Operative procedure for acute aortic dissection involving the ascending aorta. Adventitial and intimal layers of dissection are reapproximated proximally and distally. The ascending aorta is replaced by a Dacron graft. The aortic valve is replaced if necessary. (Reproduced with permission from Ref. 14.)

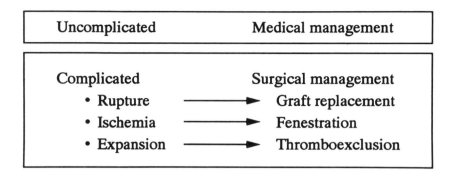

FIG. 20.10. The complication-specific approach to descending aortic dissection.

tive in restoring lower-extremity perfusion; it is usually effective as well in restoring perfusion to kidneys and intestines.

The objective of surgical treatment in descending dissection is to treat or prevent rupture and restore perfusion to vital organs; lifelong antihypertensive management is required from then on.

Postoperative Care

The preceding descriptions of the relevant surgical procedures make clear that **surgery does not cure the dissection**. Rather, **for both ascending and descending dissections, surgery is aimed at reversing or preventing life-threatening complications.** Because surgery does not eliminate the dissected aorta, postoperative care by the house officer must, as preoperatively, be directed toward the following:

1. Strictly controlling blood pressure.
2. Continuously assessing adequacy of perfusion of branch organs.

Intestinal ischemia and infarction that were not apparent preoperatively may make themselves known postoperatively. Unfortunately, this intestinal ischemia may at times take the lives of survivors of the surgical procedure.

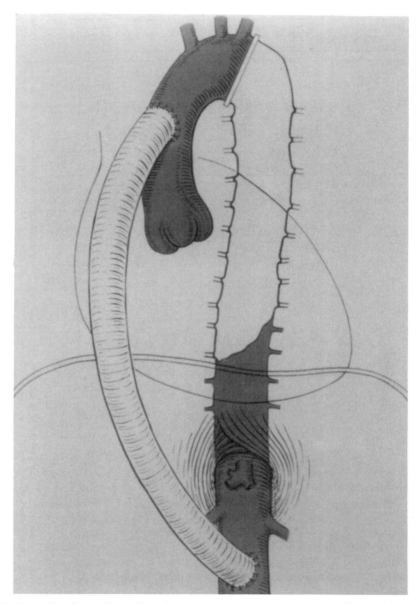

FIG. 20.11. The Carpentier, or thromboexclusion, procedure. (Reprinted with permission from Ref. 10.)

FIG. 20.12. The fenestration procedure. (Reprinted with permission from Ref. 12.)

REFERENCES

1. Tilson MD, Stansel HC. Differences in results for aneurysm versus occlusive disease after bifurcation grafts: results of one hundred elective grafts. *Arch Surg* 1980;115:1173–1175.
2. Tilson MD, Fieg EL, Harvey M. Malignant neoplasia in patients with abdominal aortic aneurysms. *Arch Surg* 1984;119:792–794.
3. Anagnostopoulos CE. *Acute aortic dissections.* Baltimore: University Park Press, 1976.
4. Najafi H. Aortic dissection. In: Sabiston DC, Spencer FC, eds. *Surgery of the chest.* Philadelphia: WB Saunders, 1983:956–967.
5. Little AG, Anagnostopoulos CE. Aortic dissections. In: Glenn WWL, Baue AE, Geha AS, et al, eds. *Thoracic and cardiovascular surgery.* Norwalk, CT: Appleton-Century-Crofts, 1983:1555–1565.
6. DeBakey ME, Lawrie GM, Crawford ES, et al. Surgical treatment of dissecting aortic aneurysms: 28 years experience with 527 cases. *Contemp Surg* 1984;25:13–23.
7. Wilson DJ, Wallen JD, Vlachakis ND, et al. Intravenous labetalol in the treatment of severe hypertension and hypertensive emergencies. *Am J Med* 1983;75 (Suppl):95–102.
8. Griepp RB, Ergin MA, Lansman SL, Galla JD, Pogo G. The physiology of hypothermic circulatory arrest. *Sem in Thorac Cardiovasc Surg* 1991;3:188-193.
9. Elefteriades JA, Hartleroad J, Gusberg RJ, et al. Long-term experience with descending aortic dissection: the *complication-specific* approach. *Ann Thorac Surg* 1992;53:11–21.
10. Carpentier A, Deloche A, Fabiani JN, et al. New surgical approach to aortic dissections: flow reversal and thromboexclusion. *J Thorac Cardiovasc Surg* 1981;81:659–668.
11. Elefteriades JA, Gusberg RJ, Kopf GS, Hammond GL, Baldwin JC. Fenestration revisited: procedure of choice for descending aortic dissection with blood flow compromise. *Arch Surg* 1990;125:786–790.

12. Haimovici H. *Vascular surgery: principles and techniques*. New York: McGraw-Hill 1976.
13. Sabiston D, Spencer F. *Gibbon's surgery of the chest*, 4th edition. Philadelphia: WB Saunders;1983.
14. Cooley D. *Techniques in cardiac surgery*. Philadelphia: WB Saunders;1984.

SUGGESTED FURTHER READING

Anagnostopoulos CE. *Acute aortic dissections*. Baltimore: University Park Press; 1976.

Now a classic, this volume recounts the unraveling of the mysteries of this disorder in a fascinating narrative by an expert in the field.

21
Additional Topics

This chapter covers a number of subjects that do not merit separate chapters but are of enough significance to warrant the house officer's awareness. These topics are therefore discussed briefly and are grouped together in a single chapter.

PROSTHETIC VALVES AND ANTICOAGULATION

Two general types of artificial heart valves are available: mechanical valves and bioprostheses. Mechanical valves are constructed from man-made materials. Bioprostheses are based mainly on biologic tissues from animals. Mechanical valves include ball valves (like the Starr-Edwards), tilting disc or "toilet seat" valves (like the Bjork-Shiley and Medtronic), and the newer double-disk valves (St. Jude). Biologic valves are mainly of two types: one type is made from glutaraldehyde-fixed porcine aortic cardiac valves mounted on a sewing ring (Carpentier-Edwards and Hancock valves); the other type uses artificial leaflets constructed from glutaraldehyde-fixed bovine pericardium (Edwards pericardial valve).

One important point is that certain **mechanical valves do not operate well at very rapid heart rates**, because poppet motion takes much more time than for normal valves. Onset of a very rapidly conducted atrial fibrillation, for example, may cause hemodynamic deterioration in a patient with a prosthetic mechanical valve.

Another point is that **a systolic flow murmur is normal following aortic valve replacement;** the prosthetic valve always creates some turbulence of flow that manifests as a murmur. (No artificial valve can re-create nature's normal laminar flow patterns.) No diastolic murmur should be audible; presence of a diastolic murmur would imply abnormal aortic regurgitation.

Likewise, no systolic murmur should be audible following mitral valve replacement; this would imply abnormal mitral regurgitation.

Mechanical valves should produce a crisp, mechanical closing sound. Loss of crispness, along with hemodynamic changes, would suggest a mechanical problem with leaflet closure. Biologic valves usually produce totally normal closure sounds.

The house officer often asks about anticoagulation practices with various prosthetic valves. Practices do vary regionally and from surgeon to surgeon. Several basic principles, however, can be enumerated.

- **In general, no anticoagulation is required in the first 48 h after surgery.** Clotting mechanisms are impaired for a period of time following cardiopulmonary bypass. Also, anticoagulation would not be safe until clot is well established at suture lines.
- **Anticoagulation is generally begun with warfarin (Coumadin) at or after the time that chest tubes are removed.** This will produce a prolongation in clotting times within 2–3 days.
- Many different schedules for coumadinization can be used effectively, as long as clotting times are followed. Some surgeons give 10 mg on the first day and 10 mg on the second and adjust according to clotting times thereafter.
- Most centers follow the prothrombin time for coumadinization, aiming for a prothrombin time about one-and-a half to two times normal. The one-and-a-half range is applied for aortic protheses and the twice normal range is used for mitral prostheses. [Remember that although the same total amount of flow passes through both the aortic and mitral valves (the cardiac output), the much larger mitral valve sees a much lower velocity of flow. The slower the velocity of blood flow, the higher the risk of thrombosis.]
- **Bioprostheses, of themselves, do not require anticoagulation, regardless of mitral or aortic position.**
- **Mechanical prostheses always require full anticoagulation with Coumadin, regardless of mitral or aortic position.**
- **Patients with a bioprosthetic mitral valve often require anticoagulation, not for the valve itself but for general cardiologic indications.** Most cardiologists would recommend anticoagulation, even without a prosthesis, for patients with mitral valve disease and atrial fibrillation, atrial thrombus, atrial dilatation, or history of arterial embolus. Most patients who come to mitral valve surgery meet one or more of these criteria.
- **Anticoagulation in a patient with a prosthetic mechanical valve should never be reversed acutely (by vitamin K or by fresh frozen plasma) without discussion with the responsible surgeon;** cases of sudden thrombosis of the mechanical prosthesis—a fatal phenomenon—have been reported with acute reversal of anticoagulation.

MAINTENANCE CARDIAC MEDICATIONS

Patients in the coronary care unit or those undergoing cardiac surgery often receive specific cardiac medications, which fall into four general categories: digitalis glycosides, diuretics, antihypertensives and afterload-reducing medications, and antianginals. The house officer must be familiar with preoperative, perioperative, and postoperative management of these drugs around the time of cardiac surgery.

Digitalis

Digitalis is usually held the morning of surgery. The operating principle is to enter surgery with the patient somewhat underdigitalized, so that digitalis toxicity, especially with potassium fluxes, is not likely. As far as the inotropy of digitalis is concerned, the much more potent intravenous agents discussed in Chapter 7 are available, if required. In fact, one cannot even appreciate clinically the mild inotropic effect of digitalis postoperatively. For control of cardiac rate, digitalis can be administered postoperatively along the paradigm discussed in Chapter 2.

Usually digitalis will be resumed as preoperatively after surgery. If digitalis was given for arrhythmia control, it is likely to be useful as part of the postoperative regimen. If digitalis was given for preoperative congestive failure, it will usually be continued for at least 6 months postoperatively. Even after successful valve replacement for congestive heart failure, some ventricular dysfunction persists. A component of dysfunction may reverse over weeks to months; a certain component may be irreversible.

Diuretics

Diuretics are usually held the morning of surgery. The reasons are several. Diuretics deplete potassium; hypokalemia is very dangerous around the time of cardiac surgery. Volume status will be monitored invasively (by CVP or Swan-Ganz catheter) and adjusted accordingly. Fluid fluxes with cardiopulmonary bypass are so massive that omitting a preoperative diuretic is largely irrelevant.

As with digitalis, patients who were on diuretics chronically preoperatively will likely be placed on them postoperatively. Again, ischemic or valvular left ventricular dysfunction that required daily diuretics preoperatively is likely to persist to some degree postoperatively.

Antihypertensives

Antihypertensive medications are usually omitted on the morning of surgery. Potent intravenous agents (discussed in Chapter 7) are available to treat intraoperative or postoperative hypertension.

Patients chronically hypertensive preoperatively will be so after recovery from surgery. At times, the specific antihypertensive drug protocol on discharge following surgery will need modification because of alteration in antianginal medications.

Table 21.1 *ACE Inhibitors*

Generic name	Trade name	Dose (mg)	Interval
Captopril	Capoten	6.25 - 50	bid - tid
Enalapril	Vasotec	2.5 - 10	bid
Lisinopril	Prinivil	10 - 40	qd
Fosinopril	Monopril	10- 40	qd

Nifedipine, a calcium antagonist with marked peripheral vasodilating properties, is very popular for acute or chronic blood pressure control. The usual dose is 10–30 mg orally four times daily.

The ACE inhibitors (angiotensin-converting enzyme inhibitors) have become extremely popular as antihypertensive agents, especially because of demonstrated beneficial effects on symptomatic state and long-term survival in patients with compromised left ventricular function. These drugs bring about peripheral vasodilation by inhibiting formation of the vasoconstrictor angiotensin II. A major toxicity is azotemia, caused by disruption of normal autoregulation of glomerular blood flow, especially in patients with underlying renal artery disease. Another toxicity is hyperkalemia, resulting from inhibition of aldosterone. Specific agents and their dosage schedules are indicated in Table 21.1.

Antianginals

Three general classes of antianginal medications are in common use: nitrates, β-blockers, and calcium antagonists. The nitrates, as discussed in Chapter 7, decrease preload, decrease afterload, and beneficially redistribute coronary flow by preventing coronary artery spasm and by dilating collateral vessels. Nitrates are available in several forms. The well-known nitroglycerin tablet is designed for emergency sublingual administration for an acute anginal attack. Many longer-acting oral nitrate preparations are available (most incorporating isosorbide). Recently, nitroglycerin paste and time-release nitroglycerin patches (lasting up to 24 h) have become popular.

Table 21.2 β-*Blockers*

Generic name	Trade name	Dose (mg)	Interval	Specific characteristics
Atenolol	Tenormin	50 - 100	Daily	Cardioselective
Metaprolol	Lopressor	50 - 200	b.i.d.	Cardioselective
Nadolol	Corgard	40 - 240	Daily	Nonselective
Pindolol	Visken	10 - 30	b.i.d.	Nonselective
Propranolol	Inderal	10 - 80	q.i.d.	Nonselective
Timolol	Blocadren	10 - 30	b.i.d.	Nonselective

Table 21.3 *Calcium Antagonists*

Generic name	Trade name(s)	Dose (mg)	Interval	Specific characteristics
Diltiazem	Cardizem	30 - 90	tid	Relatively few side effects
Nifedipine	Procardia	10 - 30	tid	Potent vasodilator; dizziness; peripheral edema
Verapamil	Calan, Isoptin	40 - 120	tid	Constipating
Nicardipine	Cardene	20 -40	tid	
Amlodipine	Norvasc	5 - 10	qd	

The β-blockers improve the oxygen supply–demand relationship in the myocardium by limiting oxygen demand; this is done through a negative inotropic effect (a decrease in strength of cardiac contraction) and a negative chronotropic effect (a decrease in heart rate). Propranolol (Inderal) is the best known of these agents. A host of newer agents have become available that may offer an advantage in cardioselectivity (causing less bronchospasm from blocking of bronchial β-receptors) or in duration of action (allowing greater spacing of doses). Table 21.2 lists the available preparations, trade names, doses, and specific characteristics of these drugs for easy reference. Each internist or cardiologist has a particular preference and usage pattern for β-blockers. Table 21.2 will allow rapid assessment by the house officer, as patients may be referred for coronary care or cardiac surgery on any of the drugs in this class. (A number of newer preparations, not yet very widely used—including acebutolol, betaxolol, carteolol, and penbutolol—are, for purposes of simplification, omitted from Table 21.2.)

The calcium antagonists improve angina through mechanisms that are not totally clear. Decrease in myocardial oxygen demand and increase in myocardial oxygen supply via coronary artery dilatation or prevention of coronary artery spasm have been postulated (1). Three calcium antagonists have been available for clinical use: diltiazem, nifedipine, and verapamil. These drugs, along with two newer ones, are summarized in Table 21.3. Again, individual cardiologists have individual preferences. Many of these drugs have become available in long-acting, sustained-release form, to allow the convenience of once-a-day dosage. (Felodipine and bepridil are omitted from Table 21.3, for simplification.)

In general, antianginals are continued up to the time of cardiac surgery, including morning doses. It has been found that abrupt withdrawal may precipitate an acute anginal attack or infarction. Also, experience has shown that cardiac surgery can be performed safely with antianginals on board. (The feared suppression of contractile function after resumption of cardiac activity post-bypass did not occur.)

At our institution, on the morning of surgery, we substitute 2 inches of nitroglycerin paste for whichever of the nitrates the patient may have been receiving. We continue the β-blocker and the calcium antagonist, generally at the same dosage. Local patterns of preoperative usage vary.

In general, after revascularization, there is no need to continue antianginals. Although a β-blocker or a calcium antagonist may be chosen to treat or to prevent supraventricular tachycardia, the indication in this setting is the arrhythmia, not angina. Also, the β-blocker or calcium antagonist medications may be required for blood pressure control, independently of their antianginal properties. A rare patient with known incomplete or inadequate revascularization may be continued on antianginals postoperatively for treatment of ischemia.

ANTIPLATELET THERAPY

There exists some recent evidence (2–4) that antiplatelet treatment may improve bypass graft patency, presumably by impairing clot formation at sites of intimal irregularity. Many cardiac surgeons routinely administer antiplatelet agents postoperatively. Aspirin and/or dipyridamole (Persantine) are prescribed for this purpose. Dosage varies from surgeon to surgeon. In one study showing a beneficial effect on graft patency, dosage was aspirin 5 gr p.o. t.i.d. and Persantine 75 mg p.o. t.i.d. In that study Persantine was begun preoperatively, and administration of both agents was implemented shortly postoperatively. Many centers have dropped the dipyridamole, using only the one aspirin tablet daily.

Many surgeons also use antiplatelet therapy postoperatively in patients who have had a bioprosthetic valve implanted. Similar dosage is used.

WOUNDS

The house officer should not instrument chest or leg wounds without discussion with more senior team members. Not infrequently, a chest wound has been needled or opened for insignificant reasons, only to lead to iatrogenic infection. A wound problem is never such an emergency that time cannot be taken to enlist an experienced opinion.

FEVER

Thermoregulation is disordered for a period of time following cardiopulmonary bypass. Almost uniformly, patients develop high fever during the first night after surgery (5). This does not signify sepsis. In fact, at our center, we do not become concerned about fevers until the third or fourth postoperative day.

NUTRITION

Most cardiothoracic patients, despite cardiac illness or undergoing major operative procedures, show little interference with gastrointestinal motility. By the morning after cardiac or thoracic surgery, most patients will be well enough to be extubated and can take nutrition orally several hours thereafter (when pharyngeal reflexes recover postextubation). Diet can usually be advanced very rapidly. Nutrition thus does not represent a problem in most patients.

An occasional patient may require prolonged ventilatory assistance or be so severely ill that oral feeding is not possible. Nasogastric feeding is used in such patients, provided that gastrointestinal motility has resumed adequately. It is important to use soft, small-caliber feeding tubes in intubated patients; **with an endotracheal tube in the trachea and a large or rigid feeding tube in the esophagus, erosion between the soft, posterior membranous trachea and the adjacent esophageal wall may result in tracheoesophageal fistula.**

It is important to start enteral feedings as early as possible, so that nutritional depletion will not be allowed to develop if the patient should require a prolonged cardiopulmonary recovery. In general, enteral feedings are preferred whenever the gut can be used; they are simple, are complete, and do not risk bloodstream infection. In unusual circumstances, a postoperative cardiac or thoracic patient may be so severely ill that gastrointestinal motility is impaired and enteral feedings are not possible. In such patients, parenteral hyperalimentation is appropriate. Many excellent reviews of this topic are available (6). Meticulous technique is imperative to avoid bacteremia, especially in patients with prosthetic cardiac valves.

RENAL FUNCTION

Renal function is so intimately related to hemodynamics that frequent reference to renal function has been made in preceding chapters. A number of key principles regarding renal functional assessment and management will be addressed specifically in this section.

Monitoring of renal function entails quantitation of urine output and measurement of blood urea nitrogen (BUN), creatinine, and electrolytes. The ICU patient will nearly always have an indwelling urinary catheter in the bladder. **An output of 30 ml/h of urine is sufficient (or 1/2 ml/kg of body weight/h for children).** This output will allow adequate excretion of waste products. Urine output at this level is evidence of satisfactory renal blood flow, which in turn indicates adequate cardiac output. If urine output falls below 30 ml/h, the cause must be sought and corrected. With oliguria below this level, elevation in BUN and creatinine and abnormalities in serum electrolytes may follow with time.

It is well recognized that oliguria can have three major physiologic causes:

1. **In prerenal azotemia, renal blood flow is insufficient.** This insufficiency may result from decreased cardiac output, which may in turn be from hypovolemia or from pump failure.
2. **In postrenal azotemia, a mechanical obstruction blocks egress of urine from the kidney.** This may be an anatomic obstruction in the ureters, bladder, or urethra; more commonly, in the ICU, obstruction occurs from mechanical occlusion of the urinary catheter by kinking, clotting, or displacement. It is wise to replace

the urinary catheter as part of the evaluation of new oliguria in the ICU patient, so that mechanical factors are eliminated as concerns. Simply irrigating the catheter for assessment of patency can be misleading.

3. **In renal azotemia, dysfunction of the kidney itself causes oliguria.** Glomerulonephritis, interstitial nephritis, and "acute tubular necrosis" are common general causes (7). Cardiopulmonary bypass, as is well appreciated, may injure the kidneys via many mechanisms (8). Renal blood flow may be reduced during bypass, especially if atherosclerotic renal artery disease preexists. Nonpulsatile flow may not be as good for the kidneys as normal pulsatile flow. Microemboli to the kidneys may occur. Hemolysis may impose a hemoglobin load on the tubules, resulting in obstruction by casts. Low cardiac output and hypotension postoperatively may further injure the kidney. For all these reasons, true renal azotemia may occur following cardiac surgery. Postoperative renal dysfunction has been shown to be more common in patients with even mild preexisting renal insufficiency (9).

Urine electrolytes and specific gravity can aid in differentiating prerenal from renal oliguria (7) (Table 21.4). In prerenal oliguria, specific gravity is greater than 1.015 and urine sodium is less than 10 mEq/liter. Urine osmolality exceeds that of plasma by greater than twofold, and urine-to-plasma ratios of BUN and creatinine exceed 20:1. Serum BUN level is more than ten times that of serum creatinine. All these relations are lost in acute renal parenchymal failure. In particular, specific gravity is low (approaching that of serum), sodium concentration is high (>20 mEq/liter), urine osmolality is less than two times that of serum, urine-to-plasma ratios of urea and creatinine are less than 20:1, and serum BUN usually does not exceed ten times creatinine.

Once the cause of the oliguria is determined, appropriate treatment can be instituted. Prerenal oliguria requires optimization of cardiac output. Postrenal oliguria requires mechanical correction. True acute renal failure may require dialysis if severe. Dialysis may be performed peritoneally, if circumstances permit; alternatively, hemodialysis is possible even shortly after cardiac surgery.

Because postoperative renal failure carries a high mortality, prevention is key. The surgeon will optimize renal protection during cardiopulmonary bypass. **The**

Table 21.4 *Urine electrolytes in oliguria*

	Prerenal	Renal
Urine specific gravity	> 1.015	<1.015
Urine sodium	< 10 mEq/liter	> 20 mEq/liter
Urine/plasma osmolality	> 2:1	< 2:1
Urine/plasma BUN Urine/plasma creatinine	> 20:1	< 20:1
Serum BUN/creatinine	> 10:1	≤ 10:1

house officer can aid in prevention by optimizing cardiac output post-operatively (thus assuring adequate renal blood flow) **and by maintaining an adequate urine output at all times** (to clear debris from renal tubules).

Recent experience (10) has shown that cardiac surgery can be performed reasonably safely even in patients with chronic renal failure requiring dialysis.

One more point deserves emphasis. Nature's response to trauma or major surgery includes an outpouring of antidiuretic hormone (ADH) and aldosterone (7). ADH promotes resorption of free water in the renal tubules, and aldosterone stimulates salt conservation. These hormones may lead to a physiologic oliguria with the electrolyte and chemistry profile of prerenal azotemia. This may occur despite adequate volume status and good myocardial function. In this setting, diuretics may be required to promote urinary flow and to prevent development of volume overload as fluids are administered.

ACID-BASE BALANCE

Every house officer has probably discovered his or her own favorite references on the topic of acid-base balance. In the ICU patient, rapid evaluation of acid-base status is needed for prompt, appropriate treatment. In this section, we provide two tools to assist the house officer in rapid acid-base assessment: (1) the acid-base rule for assessing respiratory/metabolic components and (2) the acid-base nomogram.

The Acid-Base Rule

The acid-base rule for assessing respiratory/metabolic components can help the house officer quickly determine, without tables or charts, what the respiratory component of an acid-base disturbance is. If CO_2 is normal, that is, 40 mm Hg, no respiratory component exists; any disturbance must be metabolic. **In general, for every 10 mm Hg that CO_2 rises above 40 mm Hg, pH falls 0.05.** Thus if a patient's arterial blood gases (ABGs) show pH 7.30, pCO_2 of 60, and pO_2 of 75, pCO_2 is 20 mm Hg above normal; this will drop pH by 2×0.05, or 0.10. Normal pH is 7.40, so pH would be expected to be 7.30 just from the respiratory change. This patient thus has a pure respiratory acidosis. If another patient's ABGs showed pH 7.20, pCO_2 of 60, and pO_2 of 75, the acidosis would be disproportionate even after accounting for the CO_2 rise; this patient has a mixed respiratory and metabolic acidosis.

In general, for every 10 mm Hg that CO_2 falls below 40 mm Hg, pH rises 0.10. Thus if a patient's ABGs show pH 7.60, pCO_2 of 20, pO_2 of 75, pCO_2 is 20 mm Hg below normal; this will raise pH by 2×0.10, or 0.20. Normal pH is 7.40, so pH would be expected to be 7.60 just from the respiratory change. This patient thus has a pure respiratory acidosis. If his pH were greater than 7.60, he would have a component of metabolic alkalosis as well.

This rule can be immensely valuable clinically. Respiratory abnormalities can be corrected by adjusting pCO_2 as outlined in Chapter 1. Metabolic abnormalities can be

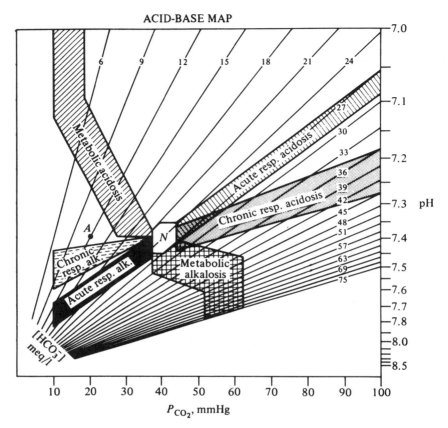

FIG. 21.1. The acid-base nomogram. (Reprinted with permission from Ref. 13.)

corrected accordingly. Metabolic acidosis can be corrected acutely by administering sodium bicarbonate. A general physiologic cause, often low cardiac output or diabetic ketoacidosis, must be sought and corrected appropriately. Metabolic alkalosis is not as common or as threatening as acidosis; usually in the cardiac patient alkalosis is of the hypokalemic, hypochloremic type that requires salt and potassium replacement. The acid-base rule, although not perfect, is accurate enough for proper clinical decision making and intervention.

The Acid-Base Nomogram

The acid-base nomogram, reproduced in Figure 21.1, **plots pH, serum bicarbonate (HCO₃), and pCO₂. On the nomogram, ranges for acute and chronic respiratory and metabolic alkalosis and acidosis are indicated.** This allows somewhat more precise assessment than the acid-base rule given earlier; in particular, the nomogram is useful for assessment of chronic states. The house officer needs merely to plot the pH, HCO_3, and pCO_2 obtained on ABG determination to ascertain to what category of acid-base abnormality a given patient's parameters usually correspond.

Practice with the acid-base rule and the acid-base nomogram will give the house officer clinical facility in the often difficult problem of acid-base assessment.

HEPARIN-INDUCED THROMBOSIS AND THROMBOCYTOPENIA

It is critically important that the house officer be familiar with the syndrome of heparin-induced thrombosis and thrombocytopenia (HITT), sometimes referred to as "heparin allergy" (11,12). Over the last several years it has become recognized that this is a common and very serious condition that can lead to devastating vascular complications. In fact, it is becoming clear that many of the patients who, prior to the recognition of this disorder, had unexplained limb ischemia or organ dysfunction actually suffered from heparin-related thrombosis.

In HITT, the patient is allergic to the administered heparin. Antibody adherence to the heparin leads to platelet activation and widespread formation of intravascular thrombus, both venous and arterial. The widespread thrombosis leads to consumption of platelets and hence to the thrombocytopenia that characterizes the disorder.

The following points deserve emphasis:

- **The development of HITT requires at least two exposures to heparin,** the first producing sensitization and the second or subsequent doses leading to the syndrome in the presence of preformed antibody.
- **Up to 10% of patients who receive heparin have an immune response and develop HITT.**
- **The severity of HITT varies widely**. The syndrome can vary from one of mild fall in platelet count without any clinical sequelae to one of widespread thrombosis, leading to venous thrombosis with pulmonary emboli and a variety of arterial thrombotic phenomena, including extremity thrombosis and limb loss, cerebral thrombosis with cerebral vascular accident, renal artery thrombosis with renal infarction and failure, hepatic artery thrombosis with hepatic necrosis and failure, and coronary artery or coronary graft thrombosis with myocardial infarction.
- **Many patients have an arterial intervention** (arterial stick, cardiac or peripheral vascular catheterization, cardiac or vascular surgery) **that triggers HITT-induced thrombosis in the involved artery.**
- **Cardiac surgical patients are especially prone to HITT**, as all have had an initial heparin exposure during catheterization and then receive massive doses of heparin for cardiopulmonary bypass.
- **Complete cessation of heparin is essential once the diagnosis is made or suspected**. No method of administration of heparin is safe, whether subcutaneous or intravenous. Switching from porcine to beef heparin is not necessarily effective. Even the small amount of heparin in the auto-flushes for arterial lines can trigger continuation of the HITT phenomenon and must be discontinued.

- The full-blown HITT syndrome carries a very poor prognosis, with a mortality exceeding 50%.
- The key to limiting the damage from this devastating disorder is keeping a high index of suspicion and making an early diagnosis. The diagnosis should be entertained in any patient who manifests a fall in platelet count on heparin therapy. The diagnosis should be suspected in any patient who develops evidence of limb ischemia unexpectedly postoperatively. The same is true for unexplained manifestations of cerebral, intestinal, hepatic, or renal ischemia.
- A platelet aggregation test is available; this test, though definitive if positive, lacks sensitivity (thought to be only about 50%). Nonetheless, the test should be ordered when the suspicion of HITT is raised.

Illustrative case: A 46-year-old male was admitted to an outlying hospital with an inferior-wall myocardial infarction in progress. He was given TPA (tissue plasminogen activator) with resolution of ischemic changes. He underwent cardiac catheterization, which revealed 95% stenoses of both the LAD (left anterior descending) and the RCA (right coronary artery). He was given continuous IV heparin. Over the next 48 h he became desperately ill, with respiratory failure and limb ischemia. He was found to have suffered multiple pulmonary emboli. He developed ischemia of three limbs, including the leg through which the catheterization had been performed. He was found to have occlusion of both femoral arteries and one brachial artery.

He underwent operative thrombectomy of both femoral arteries and the one brachial artery. He required placement of an inferior vena caval filter for repeated pulmonary emboli. He developed anuric renal failure. Thrombocytopenia had developed.

A test for heparin antibodies was positive. HITT was recognized and heparin discontinued. Coumadin was substituted. Pulmonary failure resolved, as did renal failure. Cardiac status remained stable.

The patient was transferred after recovery to our institution, where he successfully underwent coronary artery bypass, with two internal mammary artery bypass grafts, one to the LAD and one to the RCA. Anticoagulation for the procedure was achieved through the use of Ancrod (snake venom), to avoid heparin administration. This case is a vivid demonstration of the protean consequences of HITT. Many patients, especially if the HITT is not recognized, do not survive the multiple serious insults consequent to HITT. This case is described to heighten the house officer's index of suspicion regarding HITT.

A very high proportion of ICU patients currently receive heparin, which is popular for treatment of myocardial ischemia; many patients have invasive arterial catheterizations or cardiac surgical procedures; and, nearly all patients have indwelling lines that require continuous automatic heparin flushing. The house officer with a high index of suspicion will likely make a life-saving diagnosis of HITT during a year in an ICU environment.

REFERENCES

1. Feldman RL. Using calcium antagonists in rest and effort angina. *Drug Ther* 1983;(January):43–60.
2. Chesebro J, Clements I, Foster V, et al. A platelet-inhibitor-drug trial in coronary-artery bypass operations. *N Engl J Med* 1982;307:73–78.
3. Goldman S, Copeland J, Moritz T, et al. Starting aspirin therapy after operation: effects on early graft patency. *Circulation* 1991;84:520–526.
4. Gavaghan TP, Gebski V, Baron DW. Immediate postoperative aspirin improves vein graft patency early and late after coronary artery bypass graft surgery: a placebo-controlled, randomized study. *Circulation* 1991;83:1526–1533.
5. Wilson AP, Treasure T, Gruneberg RN, et al. Should the temperature chart influence management in cardiac operations? Result of a prospective study in 314 patients. *J Thorac Cardiovasc Surg* 1988;96:518–523.
6. Dudrick S, Rhoads J. Metabolism in surgical patients: protein, carbohydrate, and fat utilization by oral and parenteral routes. In: Sabiston D, ed. *Davis-Christopher textbook of surgery.* Philadelphia: WB Saunders; 1977:150–177.
7. Geha, AS. Acute renal failure in cardiovascular and other surgical patients. *Surg Clin North Am* 1980;60:1151–1166.
8. Edmunds L, Stephenson L. Cardiopulmonary bypass for open heart surgery. In: Glenn W, Baue A, Geha A, et al, eds. *Thoracic and cardiovascular surgery,* 4th ed. Norwalk, CT: Appleton-Century-Crofts; 1983:1091–1105.
9. Abel R, Buckley M, Austen W. Acute postoperative renal failure in cardiac surgical patients. *J Surg Res* 1976;20:341–348.
10. Love J. *Cardiac surgery in patients with chronic renal disease.* Mt Kisco, NY: Futura; 1982.
11. Makhoul RG, Greenberg CS, McCann RL. Heparin-associated thrombocytopenia and thrombosis: a serious clinical problem and potential solution. *J Vasc Surg* 1986;4:522–528.
12. Walls JT, Curtis JJ, Silver D, Boley TM. Heparin-induced thrombocytopenia in patients who undergo open heart surgery. *Surgery* 1990;4:686–693.
13. Rose B. *Clinical physiology of acid-base and electrolyte disorders.* New York: McGraw-Hill;1977.

SUGGESTED FURTHER READING

Walls JT, Curtis JJ, Silver D, Boley TM. Heparin-induced thrombocytopenia in patients who undergo open heart surgery. *Surgery* 1990;4:686–693.

An excellent review of the topic of heparin-induced thrombosis and thrombocytopenia; recommended for all readers, regardless of specialty.

Index

INDEX